PROSPERING WITH CANCER
SECOND EDITION

The continuing story of finding the Joyful
and
Valued Lessons that Cancer Provides

Written by Randy Chalfant, Loveland, CO.

ISBN-13: 978-1494850265

ISBN-10: 1494850265

I0439207

Front Cover Design: Randy Chalfant

Editor: Eric Boyd

Photography: Clip art, Randy Chalfant, and Jamie Hurt

Inspiration

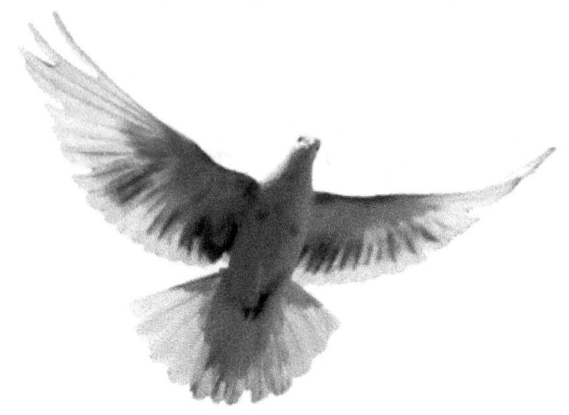

We rejoice in the hope of the glory of God. Not only so, but we also rejoice in our sufferings, because we know that suffering produces perseverance; perseverance, character; and character, hope. And hope does not disappoint us, because God has poured out his love into our hearts by the Holy Spirit, whom he has given us.

-*Romans 5*

Table of Contents

Acknowledgements

I owe everything to God, my entire life, and everything in it. God has always been with me, even when I wasn't paying attention. Cancer is an evil issue, but I believe God uses disharmony to lead one back to the flock. Cancer provided that for me, and the gift of that alone exceeds any issues caused by the disease.

I want to thank Dr. Sam Shelanski, and all of his staff for the excellent medical care they have provided. You can pay a person to do a job, money does not provide for the love, deep concern and care they so expertly, generously and happily provide.

I have been the recipient of the loving attention of more people that have befriended me than I deserve. I certainly don't feel I earned it by first giving what they abundantly gave me. Nevertheless, their constant gift of friendship was the inspiration and love that made a material difference in giving me the will to carry on through dark and difficult times.

Thanks to Eric Boyd for donating his time to edit and promote this book. Eric and I worked together, where Eric edited the technical papers I wrote. He is a rare talent that makes the process an enjoyable experience. He somehow is tuned into the spirit of what I am trying to say, and is able to always make my creative mess better. Eric is a great editor, and a great man. Thank you Eric, I truly appreciate your work.

Sue Klahr is a cancer survivor and friend. Sue called me early in my fight with cancer and gave me some insights on what to expect. It added a valuable perspective that helped me to cope with where I was and where I was going. Sue also has read this book and provided guidance. Thank you Sue, for your generosity and loving support. Your spirit exemplifies the very best of God's command to love thy neighbor, which you somehow stretched to include me.

Of course my family has been very concerned and full of loving support. Nobody really knows what the physical and emotional journey looks like unless you live with someone that has cancer. My amazing wife Bonnie has experienced every moan and groan I have had.

In ways I would never have anticipated, she has supported and cared for me. My cancer experience is in some ways more difficult for her, than it is for me. Yet, she has watched me like a hawk, sometimes sensing issues before I was really aware, and then caring for me with the love and generosity of a Saint. No complaints, and no hesitation.

Where she has found the courage to remain strong and intact I will never know. Even though she has been traumatized by all of this, she has been emotionally, spiritually, and physically a pillar of strength.

I swear, I can't do anything without her knowing and assessing it. Even in the middle of the night, if something unusual happens she is awake and tuned in, making sure nothing is going south. How does she do that?

This book is dedicated to my wife of 39 years in appreciation for a life we have shared, and for her efforts in loving and making my life happy.

Introduction

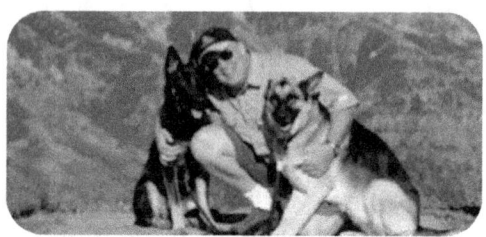

Randy, Roxy, and Gretchen

Nobody grows up thinking about the possibility of a terminal disease. We lead our lives as we do, including involvement with family, friends, school, work, and personal interests.

For many, a day comes when you learn you have cancer. Suddenly all priorities shift and you, along with everyone in your circle, are impacted.

For me, a brush with mortality crystallized the differences between what things are important, and more profoundly, what things are not important.

This book is dedicated to finding peace and joy in the process of battling cancer, and inner strength, when physical strength is all but gone.

This is the second edition of this book. While I have made some formatting changes, the bulk of the new content brings the reader up to date in the section title "Today."

Randy Chalfant

Chapter 1 - Life is Normal

"Most of the shadows of this life are caused by our standing in our own sunshine."

~ Ralph Waldo Emerson

I'm nobody special. I grew up in Colorado socially in middle America. I did know at a very early age that electronics would be my calling. I found my way through an electronic education, and moved to California to practice my trade. I soon met Bonnie at work; we were married within months, lasting some 38 years at this point. We had two children, David and Marci. We moved around chasing career carrots with Bonnie taking care of the family. We have always been campers and outdoor people. We have led a healthy life-style with no major issues.

We had, loved and cared for horses for 28 years. They lived at home with us as a part of our family. At one point I went to night school for two years at the San Jose Police academy, and eventually became a volunteer Alameda County Deputy Sheriff on a mounted division. Sr. Second Lieutenant no less!

German Shepherds could always (and still can be) found at our house and are always with us. To us they are like babies.

Whenever we moved, the whole entourage came along. That made things a bit more complicated, but the joy outweighed the effort and expense.

We have maintained the camping focus, although now it is probably more accurately described as RVing. It appeals to the outdoor calling in Bonnie and I, and the dogs. It also gives me ample opportunity to
practice my passion in photography.

In the midst of my career I thought the work I was engaged in (errantly) made me special. I was an executive, a global traveler, and as an expert in my field, frequently delivered "important" speeches to large audiences and private briefings to prestigious small groups and executives. I was also consulting with fortune 50-200 company in Information Technology (IT), saving them millions in IT costs while making millions for my company.

While I was busy in my career doing all sorts of highly visible things, my mind was focused on developing technology solutions, sales strategies, and traveling around creating large amounts of business for the companies I worked for.

It was fast paced and a constant demand. It took lots of focus and I was completely into it. I loved wheeling and dealing, doing the right things for customers, saving them money, making technology challenges easier to understand and operate, and teaching others in my organization how to do the same. It was challenging, fun, and rewarding in a worldly sort of way. But without even realizing it and because of my choices, many spiritual values and truths were hidden from me.

Something is Wrong

Stepping back from how great I felt in my personal and career-based life, maybe as far back as two years from the big event, I began to feel like something was wrong from a health point of view. My energy level was waning, and I was occasionally feeling nauseated for no apparent reason. I felt like I was too busy to pay attention to the early warning signs that were there. I'm sure it was some form of denial. One thing is certain; I would have been better off taking care of the issue then. Ignoring the signs was a mistake.

A life Changing Event

In the summer of 2010 I began working on a sales strategy that could lead to a partnership with a fortune 50 company. If won, the partnership would change the company I was working for in large and positive ways. The challenge was that although both were technology companies, they were very far apart in understanding one another and the potential symbiotic value.

I spent months developing a strategy and building presentations and spreadsheets that would bring a common understanding of how we would combine these two technologies to provide a common value.

In August of 2010 I flew to San Jose, California to meet with the partner company, along with a host of executives from other organizations. My presentation was polished, compelling and ready to go, as I was to meet with company officials the following day.

The morning of the presentation I got up to take care of routine biological business, and discovered I was bleeding... a lot. I said to myself, "yeah, I'm fine!" Got dressed, had breakfast, went to the airport to pick up the other executives from my company and drove to the big sales call.

When we got to the lobby I had the sudden urge to go the bathroom. I bled again... big. That's when I finally got the clue that it would be a good idea to go to the hospital.

I told the guys I wasn't able to complete the sales call, handed the presentation to a colleague and told them I was heading to a hospital... alone. It was definitively dumb. My colleagues were tripping over themselves to take me. But I stoically said, "nah, I have GPS. I can make it."

So I headed to the rental car on my own, set the GPS for the nearest hospital and started driving. As I drove I began feeling light headed. So I called my wife, Bonnie in Colorado. I kept her on the phone, telling her the mile makers as I passed them towards the hospital. My thinking was that if I felt faint I would pull to the side of the road. And if I passed out, Bonnie could call 911 and tell them where I was.

Nevertheless, I made it to O'Conner hospital in San Jose. I walked into emergency and told them

I had a rectal hemorrhage. They had me in the back pretty fast. They got me out of my clothes and started asking all sorts of admission and health related questions while they checked my vitals, hooked me up to a heart monitor and actually did an EKG. Thirty minutes into this entire hubbub, I had the urge to go to the toilet again. This time they put a "hat" on the toilet seat to catch what came out. It was about three pints of blood.

That seemed to get everybody excited. Doctors began arriving and discussion started about what this could be. What was being expressed to me was, "nothing to worry about. We will get this fixed. No problem".

Another thirty minutes go by, and again, I had the urge to go to the toilet. This time they also wanted a urine sample.

OK. So I go to the toilet, where they installed a fresh "hat." I again, filled it with blood. Finished with all of that, and I was taking the lid off the urine specimen jar I knew I was about to pass out. I opened the door where I could see the nurse's station directly in front of me and took a knee to avoid an uncontrolled fall. Suddenly my bed was there as they rolled it to me. I managed to stand for just a moment and collapsed onto the bed. At that point I lost my vision. I could see light, but couldn't make anything out. My hearing went. I knew there were people talking around me, lots of people and they were talking fast, but I couldn't understand anything. In time my vision slowly came back as did my hearing. I then learned that I had "crashed", they had nearly lost me. My blood pressure had dipped to around 40/15. The seriousness of the tone among the doctors and nurses took a dramatic step up at that point.

I was admitted into the hospital and taken to an area that is just below intensive care and is known as critical care. They connected me to bio monitors for 24-7 observation from a nearby station. There was constant attention.

They put a wheel chair by my bed so I could get to the bathroom, as I was soon too weak to walk.

The hemorrhaging went on all day. The plan was that if the bleeding didn't stop by 6pm, they would do a colonoscopy and cauterize whatever was bleeding. I was really concerned. I didn't want to wait. I was anxious to take care of it. They also did a CT scan (Formerly known as a CAT scan - Computerized Axial Tomography) to see what was happening. But that didn't drive them to any major conclusions, other than they could see there was a tumor.

At 8pm I requested they do *something*, as every thirty minutes I was bleeding out. They were noncommittal. Which was odd because they were constantly taking blood samples and could see that my red blood cell count was falling off the cliff. A normal red blood cell count should be above 14. Mine was at 8 and falling. Eventually it went below 7. I had lost half my blood supply!

Time to take action! I talked to the floor nurses – noncommittal. I called to talk to the hospital administrator. I told them they had thirty minutes to take care of me or I was calling for an ambulance to take me to a hospital that would treat me. That got the ball rolling. They did the colonoscopy. They also took a biopsy of the tumor they found and cauterized to stop the bleeding. I was calling Bonnie at home every time some news arrived. She wanted to immediately get on a plane and come, but I told her not to.

Too complex to take care of the dogs and expensive to get and stay there, I felt it was unnecessary and it would have been too much expense. I felt like I could handle the situation and get home.

A Gripping Discovery

I had lost nearly half my blood supply that Friday, and discovered I had a tumor in my rectum. Saturday, the attending physician talked about the likelihood of Cancer. She told me the biopsy showed Cancer tendencies although they were not certain. Hearing the word "Cancer" caused my whole body to physically tighten as I was instantly gripped by fear.

I didn't hear too much of what else she had to say. Cancer. Me? I've got Cancer? I'm going to die? I'm going to suffer though some horrible regimen of treatments that makes me feel like I am dying, and then die anyway? "OK. Deep breathe. Calm down." In that moment I realized this is bigger than me. And I turned to God and prayed. "Heavenly father, this is too much for me to handle, I am turning it over to you. I am freeing myself from fear and worry, and I will have faith that you will take care of me as you have always done." That was probably the single smartest decision of my life.

The Beginning of Grace

Thursday, the night before all of the trouble began, I had called a dear friend, John Tomasetti, who lives in Palo Alto, just to say hello. It turned out that he happened to be in Denver for some work he was doing. When Saturday morning arrived, I thought I would let him know about the ordeal and the news I had received. I also knew it would be comforting to talk to him. He of course was shocked by the news. Minutes later, I got a call from his bride, Deborah, who said she was coming down to see me. I, of course, told her that it wasn't necessary. But being the saint that she is, she showed up anyway. I realized how kind it was. When John got home Saturday, he brought over a large folder of DVD movies for me to keep myself entertained. Boy, wasn't that nice?

They wouldn't release me Saturday, because of how weak I was and that fact that my heart was racing up to 140 to 165 BPM every time I stood up due to the lack of blood. The concern was that it would create a heart attack. They kept trying to give me a blood transfusion, which I consistently refused. They asked if I had religious objections, I told them no. Truthfully, I don't have much faith in the advances in screening and cleaning methods.

Reluctantly, they did release me Sunday. John insisted on taking me to the airport. It was so kind. He wheeled me around in the wheelchair because I couldn't walk.

It was just the beginning of what I found to be an avalanche of people searching for a way to do something to express their love, concern, and desire to do something for me. It was the seed that opened into a much larger revelation and understanding of the abundant love and generosity of humankind. I will address this in much more detail later.

What's important here is that I saw something that was always around - for the first time. Prior to that point it had been seemingly invisible to me. I take responsibility for being too full of myself and caught up in things that are most often considered important on a worldly measuring scale.

Medical Challenges

I managed to fly home on Sunday, but it was a serious physical challenge. The pilots were on notice for alternate landing places in case of a medical emergency. United gave me a first class seat to recline in, because I couldn't physically tolerate sitting straight up. The flight attendants were fussing over me constantly to make sure I had everything I needed.

The first thing they did was to give me a liter bottle of water. They brought me a blanket because I was cold, served food to me first... just anything and everything possible. God Bless them. That never happens! They had a wheelchair waiting at the plane door. They wheeled baggage claim then down to where Bonnie was waiting to pick me up.

We knew when we got home that I was too weak to stand the greeting that my special love (Roxy, my beloved German Shepherd) would give me. So, I waited in the garage while Bonnie let her out to go potty. Once Roxy was out, I made it to the bedroom, took off my clothes and got into bed. When Bonnie let her back in, Roxy hesitated at the back door, sensing someone else was in the house. On guard, she went first, into the formal dining room to gain visual advantage of who was in the bedroom. When I saw her, I called her name. She cried, ran and leapt onto the bed crying, squealing, spinning, falling down on me, up again, down again, and massive puppy kisses on the face. True love.

Monday I went in to see my family physician. He looked at me for about five minutes, and asked if I would like an ambulance, or if Bonnie would be taking me to the hospital. I didn't need the drama of an ambulance, so Bonnie took me over to the hospital. But, my doctor personally wheeled me to the car.

So it was over to Medical Center of the Rockies in Loveland. They kept me. The first thing that came up was a transfusion. I told them I didn't want blood, and no, it isn't a religious objection. They patiently explained why blood was safer today than in the past and that I needed it. I still refused on Monday.

That afternoon, a staff surgeon, Dr. Joe Livengood came in to give me an exam, and talk about the results of the biopsy. He is a very caring and intelligent man, however he wasn't pulling any punches. He laid it out graciously and straight. He believed that I have Cancer, and it needed to be cut out. He spent at least an hour in my room talking to me. Oddly. I was OK with all of it.

When he left a nurse immediately came in. She asked if I was OK. I thought that was strange, I said I was fatigued but fine. It turns out she was there because most people when they hear they have Cancer, have a large emotional melt down. I didn't. Why not? Because I passed the baton to God early on and from that point forward I was simply a passenger on a bus. I knew there were going to be bumps, but I am trusting God to drive me safely through.

The doctors and Bonnie ganged up on me on Tuesday afternoon. I finally gave in and took the blood transfusion they were all fussing about. Oddly enough, I instantly felt better (duh). My strength returned to the extent I could stand up, so I got dressed to leave.

Just as I was leaving, the doctor that had argued with me to take the transfusion came into the room. I walked right up to her, put my arm around her and said, "I'm not going to tell you I feel better". We had a good laugh, a nice hug, and I left to go home.

Within a week I had met with Dr. Livengood again. We discussed surgical options, but he wanted to really understand what we were dealing with. He scheduled a colonoscopy, which included ultrasonography. The two big objectives were a better biopsy and to discover if in fact it is malignant and the depth of invasion of the intestinal cancer.

The procedure confirmed that it was stage 2A rectal cancer. Stage 2A, colon cancer signifies that the cancer has migrated into the muscle layers of the rectum, but importantly, has not made it outside of the rectum to other surrounding tissue, and no lymph-node involvement.

The bad news is that the location of the cancerous tumor is too low to be operable. Ordinarily surgeons would just cut it out, or partially remove the rectum and resect it. In my case that isn't possible, unless they do a colostomy, which they call an Abdominal-Perineal Resection (APR), which I have refused. As such, the only option is either chemo or radiation.

As a result, I was sent off to an oncologist. That's when I met Doctor Sam Shelanki. Dr. Shelanki came walking into the treatment room the first time in a button-up shirt, blue jeans, and expensive cowboy boots and introduced himself as Sam. I liked him immediately. The plan was to go to radiation. He set me up at the hospital to get radiation . . . no chemo.

On a visit to the hospital to set the scanners for targeting, I met with a radiologist. He was looking at my CT scan from California a few weeks earlier. He had found some spots on my lungs. I told him to not worry about that, they were caused by a spore I had picked up in Australia and my lungs would always look that way. He said, "that's very interesting. I'm setting you up for a _Positron Emission Tomography_ (PET) scan immediately."

The test involves injecting a very small dose of a radioactive chemical, called a radiotracer, into the vein of the arm. PET scans are most commonly used to detect cancer. The tracer is basically a nuclear-doped sugar. Since cancer is based on fast growing tissue, sugar is drawn to cancer sites as necessary energy used for tissue growth.

The Tomography part of the PET scan, is just like a CT scan. This provides a 3D view of the body or scanned area. The Positron Emission part, has to do with the half-life of the nuclear doped sugar. As the short half-life is reached, the radiotracer throws off positrons. There are sensors in the PET machine that can see, and locate where they come from. That added to the Tomography and they can see activity levels of fast growing cells, exactly where they are located, how large they are, and how active they are. This is a major blessing in understanding cancer in your body and what to do about it.

One of the main differences between PET scans and other imaging tests like CT scan or MRI is that the PET scan reveals the cellular level metabolic changes occurring in an organ or tissue. This is important and unique because disease processes often begin with functional changes at the cellular level. A PET scan can often detect these very early changes whereas a CT or MRI detect changes a little later as the disease begins to cause changes in the structure of organs or tissues.

Fear. . . and lots of it

After the PET scan, Bonnie and I went back in to see Dr. Shelanki, or Sam, as you quickly become on a first name basis with the people who are caring for you through such a personal ordeal. Sam gave us the results of the PET scan. It appeared that the spots on my lungs also looked like cancer, which would move me from stage 2A to stage 4, meaning the cancer had spread to a different location or metastasized.

Then Sam dropped the bomb, and told Bonnie and I that if it is metastatic lung cancer, it is incurable. Terminal cancer. Statistically, I had a year to a year and a half to live (most probably), with five years on the outside. You can imagine, it was hard news for Bonnie and I. It was a difficult moment.

He ordered a biopsy scan, "STAT" (medical terminology for immediate), meaning – no kidding - right now! Bonnie and I drove straight to the hospital, where doctors used a long needle guided by a CT scanner to reach a tumor site through my back where they could take a biopsy from my lung.

Within an hour they confirmed that the colon cancer had, in fact, moved to my lungs. The doctor who took the biopsy kindly told me I was stage 4. When Bonnie came into the recovery area I told her. It was like getting news of a death sentence. Holding it together emotionally was extremely difficult in that moment. But somehow we did. Whether we were in shock, simply prepared or completely immersed in the grace of God and the love we have for each other, there was a profound calm between Bonnie and I as I got dressed and we headed home together.

So in classic medical style the worst picture was painted. The word was this is terminal and I had a year and a half to live... five years if I beat the odds.

I knew then that I would work to do better than that. I know that God is looking out for me and has blessed me with a strong positive and thankful attitude. That attitude would soon start to grow.

The Emotional Impact

I have to say; going to bed that night, where meaningful conversations often occur, was tough. That's where we would discuss the prospects for the future. The prospect now was I had no future. Bonnie and I were feeling shattered. We didn't dwell on it excessively. After all, it is what it is. But after 36 years together (at that time), it was tough to think about and more difficult to talk about.

My prayers took a quantum leap forward. I had turned it over to the Lord early on. But my tension level was greatly reduced from that point forward.

I had faith that whatever the outcome, it was being managed by and executed as a part of God's plan. Even then I knew that there are no mistakes in God's plan it was my job to be a faithful soldier and follow. It also became clear that there are two mindsets for this; one is the worldly view as seen by people; and the other is the spiritual view as seen by the Lord.

I knew that in my prayer God would never appear before me, or give me an audible answer to my deep fears and concerns. On the other hand, not one prayer has gone unanswered. Solutions have always and continue to arrive quickly and seem to address each prayer's topical issue. The more that happened, the more relaxed I became.

Chapter 2 - Working and Chemo

"A tree is known by its fruit." - Matthew 12:33

The world around you does not stop just because you have cancer. Nor did my responsibilities as the breadwinner that keeps the family running.

Fortunately, I have never carried a lot of debt. The prospects were simple; I could lose 40% of my income by going on disability, or keep working. At that particular time, losing 40% would have been difficult on us. I didn't even consider it. I was going to carry on.

Which brings up a critically important point. Having a positive mental attitude is the most important contributor to recovery and health.

To make this point, Sam, my Oncologist, told me that he had another patient that came to him with the exact same issues as me. He was stage 4 with the same metabolic issues. When Sam gave him the news that it was terminal the results for him were very different. This man went home, put on a suit, laid down on his bed, and within four hours he had passed away. He had willed himself to death! Yes, you can do that. It begs the question do you want to live or die... and for what reasons?

I believe in our Lord Jesus Christ, our Heavenly Father, the Holy Spirit, and eternal life. In fact, it sounds so good to me that in truth I would rather be there than here. But two things come to mind; 1) God's plan is not up to me. I can't presume to understand it, nor do I believe for the most part should I try, and 2) I certainly accepted a large set of responsibilities here on Earth, and I have never avoided any of them - I wasn't about to start.

My family needs me, and I want them more than I want to enjoy the glory of being in the presence of the Lord. My obligation is to carry on. *Especially* if I am terminal. I have many new goals to accomplish to ensure my family is taken care of in my absence. The first and most important thing was to continue to work to give myself time to accomplish that.

Fortunately I worked from my home office. I was writing many technical Information Technology white papers, sales strategies, developing presentation material to be used with customers, and developing strategic alliances with key partners. All of which, I could do from home.

So now I had two masters to serve. One, the job; the other, my health care.

Part of the plan was to sell the house, shed the small mortgage, and buy a new home for cash. That was the most important element in taking care of my responsibilities. Without the mortgage I could live on disability. So we started sprucing the place up for sale.

Working and doing these mental exercises was physically difficult at times. But I also found that working kept me from thinking about how I felt.

If I were to simply stop, I'd have lots of time to sense how lousy I felt. While working and staying focused on tasks I seemed to stop thinking about my discomfort.

Telephone calls, and webcasts were frequent in my career. These things would always give me a natural hit of adrenaline. People were often amazed at how good I sounded and how well I was handling the workload. My boss was astounded at the work I was producing. Her husband had died two years earlier of colon cancer, so she was familiar with what I was going through. That was also a blessing, as she was empathetic. Even so, I maintained a consistent work ethic.

It was good for me, because it made me feel good about what I was doing and the results I was achieving. It made me feel "normal" (although I've never in my life been accused of being "normal"). And at the same time it kept me distracted from how I felt.

There were certainly times while taking chemotherapy that I had to take a nap during the day, or just rest. I was generally in bed by 6pm, simply exhausted from the effort. I would turn on the TV, which was an instant formula for narcolepsy. Later, around 10pm, I would turn the lights and sound off and go to sleep again. I have found that rest is critically important. Allowing my energy to drop below a certain point always results in punishing illness.

A big part of staying able and upbeat is managing energy. I must say too, there is a thin line. Too much rest, and no physical output are nearly as bad. I have taken walks daily with my baby, Roxy – my German Shepherd along with Bonnie and her baby – Abby, another German Shepherd, even while wearing a chemo pump.

Sometimes it feels like walking through deep water and the effort it takes is immense. But I do it because I refuse to become inert.

Chapter 3 - Treatment Begins

"Sometimes the Spirit sees what is invisible to the eye."

As a result of the discovery of Stage 4 cancer, the fact that the colon cancer had moved to my lungs and the terminal nature of it, the health plan changed. Radiation was cancelled and I was to begin a chemo regimen. Oddly, I don't have lung cancer; I have colon cancer – a particular cellular structure - in my lungs.

The medical types needed an efficient way to infuse the chemicals into my body. So, on October 4th 2010 I went back to Dr. Joe Livengood to have a 'port' installed in my chest. As I was walking into the hospital, a great guy and former colleague, Joel Brunson called. He was concerned about the news he had heard, and in his typical style, spent time with me to help "pump-up" my attitude. Another generous moment, by a gracious and concerned friend.

My Super Port

It seems that everyone in chemotherapy has a port installed. A port consists of a reservoir compartment (the portal) that has a silicone bubble for needle insertion, with an attached plastic tube (the catheter).

The device was surgically inserted under my skin in my upper left chest and appears as a bump under my skin below my left clavicle. The catheter runs from the portal and was surgically inserted into my superior vena cava. The catheter terminates in my superior vena cava, just upstream of my right atrium or near my heart. This position allows infused agents (like chemo) to be spread throughout my body quickly and efficiently.

The procedure was done in the operating room. On the way to recovery, my heart rate spiked to 164 beats, which got the team pretty excited. They tried a number of drugs to get my heart rate down. None of them worked. They decided the catheter was tickling my atrium and causing the elevated heart rate. So, back to the operating room to move the catheter out of my heart.

It didn't work. They did an EKG and found a heart arrhythmia. An anesthesiologist put me out again and they defibrillated my heart to get it back in sync.

It took all of that Monday and Bonnie stayed with me the whole time for support.

Drugs . . . and lots of them

Wednesday October 6th 2010 Chemo started

I found that the amount of calls and email was becoming onerous for the level of energy I had. The only effective way to broadly keep all my friends and family informed was to write a blog. It takes some effort. But I've found that staying connected with the people by any means possible is extremely important to survival and appreciation of life while doing it. The blog can be found at www.randychalfant.com. Look for "How's Randy?"

The blog expresses, not only what is going on at the time, but also how I felt about it. It provides a real-time view of my mental state as treatment progressed. As I share some of these blogs with you here, you will notice early on, how I was focused on the treatment and how I was responding to it. But later, because of the avalanche of kindness delivered by family, and friends, there was a serious impact on me amounting to nothing short of a revelation in understanding the abundantly generous spirit of human kind. The lord Jesus added a commandment before his crucifixion which can be found in John 15:12, "This is what I tell you to do: Love each other just as I have loved you." Evidently a good part of humanity believed in the word of God, because it was poured out to me generously.

Here are some Blog posts from early on:

Wednesday, October 6, 2010
Today at 11am the real battle began.

Chemo for four hours in the oncologist's office, followed by wearing a pump, that will be filling me with F5U chemo 24 hours a day until Friday.

I am basically feeling OK, specifically I am not feeling sick per se, but I am tired.

I am working, and intend to continue to work. I love my job, company, and the team I work with.

I am not going to give up or give in. I won't be starring at the ceiling; I will be working and carrying on as I work to get through the bumps ahead.

Bonnie and I are planning for the worst and hoping for the best. She is doing OK also, although the situation is stressful for both of us at times.

I am humbled by the massive amount of calls, cards, and email I have received. I have been told how much I am loved more in the last two weeks than I have been in my entire life. Thank you. The support and care from so many is appreciated more than words can convey.

The offers for any help whatsoever for Bonnie or I is unbelievable. People are offering to bring meals, hold my hand while I am getting Chemo, a shoulder to cry on, a person to talk to, mow my lawn, anything I can think of. One friend, Brian Bate, even brought me holy water from Mexico.

How can I thank all of you? It is impossible, but thank you.

I will update this Blog to let you know things that happen.

Thursday October 7th, 2010 – So Far so Good

Well I had the big jolt of chemo yesterday, and I am wearing a pump that continues to push poison into me until tomorrow.

Feeling OK, however. Working on a presentation for my boss, conference call with Gartner, a call from a Systems Engineer on account strategy, and a conference call with my team on solutions and Web design. On the personal front, a few calls from concerned friends.

Just had soup and a sandwich and I am feeling tolerable.

I should find out on the 20th if I am a candidate for a bioengineered drug that is targeted for cancer. If I am, that should be a big enhancer to winning.

Thursday October 7th, 2010 – Touched and Humbled

It is difficult to know what the impact is that you may have on the lives of others, unless some compelling event motivates people to tell you. This may seem obvious, but telling people you may be facing death is one of them.

I am just so touched and humbled by the non-stop calls, cards, flowers, and email I am receiving. Oh yeah, somebody is sending Soup according to an email notice we just received.

Kind and good people are sending email and calling from all over the United States and in fact, the world. I could have never estimated or predicted what a positive impact it has caused inside of me. Really, who would know, unless you experience it? It is just an unbelievable experience of support, loving concern, and well wishes.

I hope someday I can return the feeling that all of you have given me. There can be no greater gift; I thank all of you humbly and gratefully.

Friday, October 8, 2010 – Strange … OK, That's Weird

I got the big dose of chemo Wednesday. They put a pump on me to get 48 continuous hours of poison.

I had the pump taken off at noon today. After the pump came off, I started to feel ill. Seems like I should have felt that way while being poisoned. Mhhhh?

The email and cards continue to come in from the corners of the planet. There is no end to the heart, love and support of good people.

A Little Discovery

What I didn't know at the time was that the steroids given as a premedication before chemo help to pump you up and make you feel better. However, they wear off about the same time the chemo pump is coming off, at which point you crash. I always feel lousy by Friday afternoon. It gets worse through Saturday. By Sunday night I would start to come around to feeling a bit better. And by Monday I was good enough to work. It wasn't easy, but I was able to manage it.

Monday, October 11, 2010 - Unexpected and Welcome

After a weekend where I could have described myself as worthless, I finally felt good today. First time I have felt decent since the end of August.

I guess this may be how it works. Get Chemo, feel crumby for 5 days, and then feel OK again. I can handle that. In fact I haven't had anything thrown at me yet I can't handle. I find that very encouraging!

Had some dear friends stop by Sunday. Mike and Ruth Cook. Bonnie and I have known them from the time we were married 36 years ago.

They brought gifts! Lunch from Mimi's Cafe, and some holy water from New Mexico. I promptly drank it! That's two varieties of holy water I have had now. Hope one or both works!

Sunday, October 17, 2010 – Patience and Looking ahead

Last week was good. I worked on some fairly demanding things with good results. Had one day that I had to knock off early to rest, but did well all of the rest.

Next Wednesday I will experience my second round of Chemo. Chemo is cumulative, so it could be that I will find the next round more challenging than the last. Have to wait and see.

I am finding this to also be a test of patience. I am certainly not used to, nor do I think I can ever become used to, not feeling well, and being able to do whatever I want whenever I want. That is a strong motivator to heal!

It is better to keep my eye on the results of healing, not the issues of the illness.

My son David flew up this weekend from New Mexico just to hang out. So nice to have him here. Kim, his wife, was unable to accompany David because of job demands. We miss seeing her, nobody to harass me! A few years ago she sent me a lump of coal for Christmas. She said I had been bad! I kept it as a treasured gift.

Marci is here for the weekend as well. Feels so good to have the kids home.

I am both looking forward to beginning treatment next week to get closer to recovery, and dreading the expected physical challenge. My commitment to healing is strong.

Thanks for the flow of cards, email and calls. They are motivating and touching.

Tuesday, October 19, 2010 – Round 2, We shall See

I saw my oncologist today for a short while. I had to have another blood draw, so they can insure the chemo dosage I get tomorrow is calibrated appropriately.

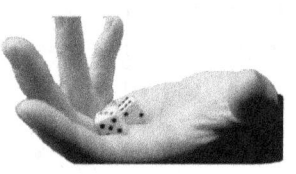

*I described how my body reacted from the first chemo treatment. The Doc was encouraged that things are going well, very well. About five weeks from now I will go in for another Positron Emission Tomography (**PET**) scan, which will tell the story for how well I am responding. Of course I would like to know now, but will once again have to exercise patience.*

I found out today that my body is not compatible with a genetically engineered treatment. One less arrow in the quiver.

Knowing how I will react to the next treatment is a roll of the dice, but most indicators are that I will do fine.

I realized today in responding to a friend in Toronto, that while my body is seriously ill, I on the other hand, am just fine. My mind will lead this effort, my body will follow.

I continue to receive calls, cards, and email daily. I am far beyond my ability to adequately express my gratitude, nevertheless - thanks for a gift of meaningful support I value with my life. I never could have predicted the outpouring this would create. Truly amazing.

Thursday, October 21, 2010 Ding! Winning Round 2

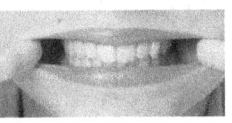

Got Chemo-Charged yesterday, and feel no worse than last time, which is completely manageable. Kind of like a low grade flu, just makes me feel low. On the other hand, I have had two conference calls this morning, and expect to complete edits on about eight solutions briefs, and complete a white paper outline. The job gives me focus. I love Nexsan, which gives me joy. You could not work for a better company, with better products, or with a better team of people. Aces.

Still haven't seen anything thrown my way I can't handle. Not trying to be cocky, more a statement of relief, and my growing confidence.

Speaking of which, my confidence grows in the belief that I will win.

Rumors of my impending death are greatly exaggerated.

Sunday, October 24, 2010 - Poisoning Your Body can make you ill

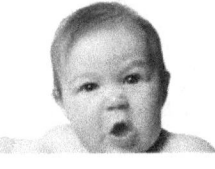

Remember the post - "OK, that's weird" from Oct 8th? I mentioned that I started feeling lousy after the Chemo was stopped. I found out that the reason for that is coincident with when the steroids fizzle out. They start chemo with an IV of steroids to keep me feeling good. They last 48 hours, which is about when the pump comes off. So, at the end of the 48 hours - kaboom, I was ill for the weekend.

Not horribly as in some stories I have heard, but still not great either.

Still, everyone around me, family, friends, and doctors are all impressed with how I am getting through this. My confidence remains high.

5 weeks from now the PET scan will tell the story. I can't wait.

This week, my Team from Nexsan sent me a Sony PSP to keep me entertained. It has turned into a serious blow to my ego. I have found that any eight-year old can whoop me.

My neighbor Pat, the best pal and neighbor God could create destroyed her fingers in making me a beautiful Afghan to keep me warm. It is seriously beautiful, soft and cozy. Bonnie is modeling it!

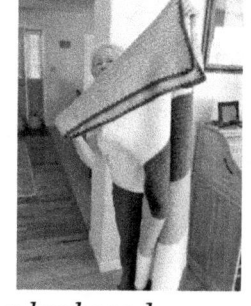

Finally, thanks to Jamie Hurt, who sent me an emergency colon, which came in the form of a colon key from a keyboard suspended in a gel inside of a jar. It provided a belly laugh of entertainment.

Evidently it was the cookie fairy that just left a batch of unbelievable chocolate chip pan style cookies on the front porch - thanks.

Sunday, October 31, 2010 - Not as good as I thought

It's so strange. How I am, depends on the moment. I can wake up feeling reasonably good, by noon feel like I need serious rest, by mid afternoon 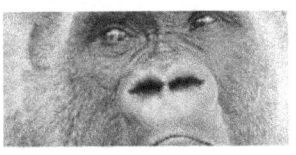 *be OK - up - down, left right - who knows. It's annoying. Imagine that issue for a type "A" personality. Argh!*

Nevertheless, Friday I drove the Vette to Boulder where I attended a client meeting, I enjoyed it so much! Among other things, I attended a competitive storage vendor's sales presentation. There was a really bright young man that did a terrific presentation. I got to ask difficult questions, to help keep it real. For me, it was as much fun as a good sporting event.

That could be a business - helping clients distinguish the difference between vendor hype and reality, and whether the value being sold by the vendor, has any measurable value to the client. Make money, and feel good about doing the right thing - I like that idea. If I weren't having so much fun working for Nexsan, I would consider that.

Saturday, I managed to change the oil in the John Deere tractor, put a new diesel fuel filter in the Jeep Liberty, vacuumed and cleaned it, went out for some carry out, and them boom, I was down. By night fall better again - up - down - left, and right.

By the way, I had another business idea. I am going to place an ad on eBay. I will explain that I have terminal cancer with a short expected life span. As such, I am selling my abilities to become a messenger. I will offer to take messages from the living to the dearly departed for a fee. Four things will happen, 1) A variety of morons will give me money; 2) The news will pick it up; 3) Some people will love me and some people will hate me; 4) The people that already know me will laugh until the cry and I will have a wad of cash to laugh over as well. What do you think? Comments are welcome.

Past my overactive sense of humor, in a month I will find out if we are killing the cancer. This isn't easy, but it isn't horrible either - so far so good.

I am grateful for the continuing flow of support from all of you. Saying thanks isn't adequate - but thanks.

Oh - and one depressing issue. Remember the Sony PSP my team from Nexsan gave me? I am finding that my ineptitude in operating the device as compared to any child to be depressing - for sure fun, but depressing.

Keep smiling.

Tuesday, November 2, 2010 - Here I go again and halfway through!

Got to the top of the roller coaster today, and start the fall back down tomorrow with the third round of

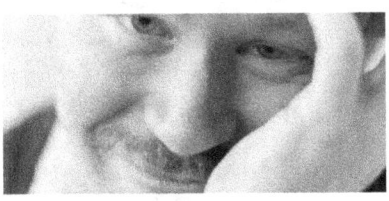

chemo. While I am certainly not looking forward to that, it is still one step closer to completing this regime. Who knows what will happen, but I remain hopeful that one regiment will serve to knock the cancer back to hades.

In the meanwhile, I had the pleasure of a visit from two near and dear friends today. They drove up from Boulder to visit. We spent too much time talking about me, because they wanted to know the whole story. I hope I can see both of them soon to spend no time on me, and all available time talking about what they are doing.

But, even though the conversation was biased toward me, it really touches me that friends really want to understand. Beyond wanting to understand the issues of the disease, everyone seems to want to know how I am handling it.

The largest impression seems to come from people not finding anger, depression, fear, defeat, or whatever. I am sure that we are all different, and it is difficult to know how any one of us will react to stressful situations, especially when it involves life or death.

However, I am confident in God's plan and believe it all makes sense. With that said, why should I worry? I am simply trying to understand what all of this is about. Maybe someday I will have the opportunity to make the journey through this path a little easier for someone else, as all of you have helped me.

So thanks for coming by Mark and Barba - I love and appreciate both of you.

Wednesday, November 3, 2010 - How was Chemo today?

I wouldn't want to leave you with the wrong impression or anything, but there are probably better ways to spend the day.

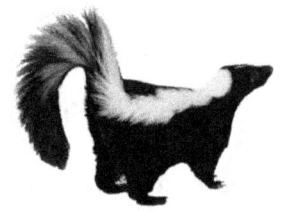

On the plus side of things, my Oncologist is beginning to say very positive and encouraging things about my future, based upon his clinical observations.

This is new. It means that he has had a chance to see how I am responding to treatment, and things are looking good.

Still three weeks from the PET scan, which will tell the story, but for the first time since this speed bump came up, I am getting good news. Keep your fingers crossed, and the prayers coming folks. I'm climbing out of this hole.

Saturday, November 6, 2010 - Getting the Vette Ready for Winter

Woke up feeling ill from coming off the chemo yesterday. Bonnie made a great breakfast with her 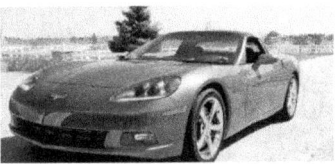 *world famous waffles. That really helped my energy come up. It is just a beautiful day, and I just couldn't stand sitting around anymore. So, I took the Vette out to the car wash, hand washed it, vacuumed it out, and changed the oil. It is now ready for winter!! On the way home I stopped by to see some friends, the McCrimmon brothers, I call 'em the Mac Boys. They run a business here in Loveland, and feel like family. It was so nice to see them.*

The whole morning had me so distracted I forgot about how I felt. Perfect. It really helps to stay engaged with work and play, and not get to focused on the issues.

When I got home, I looked at my email, and had a long and enjoyable email from another person I think the world of, John McArthur. John claims he is getting rejected from adding comments, if anyone else is noticing that let me know and I will try to figure it out. Anyway thanks for the email John, it was nice.

Finally my sister called from Lebanon where she and her husband are on vacation visiting ruins, and local attractions.

All in all - pretty nice day folks.

Wednesday, November 10, 2010 - Truth be Known

For those of you that know me, you know that I am a positive and upbeat sort of guy. I guess that is just how I am gratefully 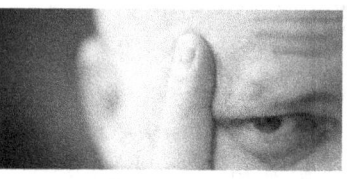 *wired. I started thinking about this BLOG, and the tone of the commentary I have written here. I am pleased with the upbeat nature of it, it resonates with the person I am.*

On the other hand, it may also not give a realistic view of what the journey is, as a result of having cancer. I won't write about all the aches and pains or the experience of being ill, frankly I find it quickly boring and I don't like being or want to become self absorbed.

However, I will say this - just to balance the record, I am ill, and it is not easy to carry on. I struggle with it daily. Some days are better than others, and some are just not good. Enough said.

I nevertheless remain excited about my work. It gives me focus, and satisfaction, which beats the day lights out of paying close attention to cancer and it's issues.

I also remain positive that I will get through this and be healthy again.

Thanks for the continuing flow of email, cards, and gifts, the love and support are the best medicine in the world.

Continuing generosity, Wendy knitted a skullcap to keep my baldhead warm - perfect timing sweetie!

Camberley sent an mp3 player/book titled Faith, Hope, and Healing. Thanks ladies - love you both.

There is no payment possible for me to return what all of you have given me. I will never forget.

Saturday, November 13, 2010 - My Wicked Humor

I had the fortune of having a breakfast meeting yesterday at the Egg and I with two colleagues/friends. We were drinking coffee and engaged in some lively conversation.

A nice young waitress approached the table and asked, "Do you need a few more minutes"? Without thinking I replied, "I was thinking I need a few more years!" She cocked her head 3 degrees starboard with a quizzical look, and the three of us burst out laughing. She walked away.

Hysterical.

Tuesday, November 16, 2010 - Oh, it's Chemo time again...

I can't say I am looking forward to tomorrow. Just about the time I start feeling reasonable, I have to get poisoned again. Whoever said medicine was tasteful? Nobody!

Talked to the oncologist today, he was again positive that things are coming along. He will schedule a PET scan sometime soon, so we will see objectively in the near future how I am really doing.

I'm going to add a countdown timer on the landing page when I know when it happens. The shell is there now.

I have learned that there is tired, and then there is chemo tired. I am the latter. While I feel beat up at the end of the day, I am still able to focus and work. I wrote a 17-page analysis today. That takes focus, and it also is something that I really enjoy.

I am very anxious to get this behind me.

If anyone is thinking I need another gift, please send baseball bat - there goes my wicked humor again.

Scott - thanks for the Corvette Book!

More soon . . .

Thursday, November 18, 2010 - Ding! Round 4 - I am still here and WINNING!! What did you expect?

Chemo definitely is enough to make you ill.

However, I am doing fine and I ran across this quote, which really resonated with me.

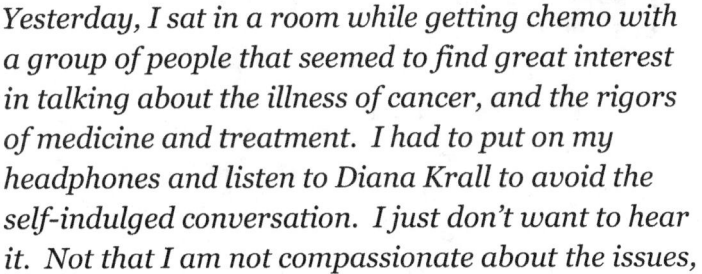

Yesterday, I sat in a room while getting chemo with a group of people that seemed to find great interest in talking about the illness of cancer, and the rigors of medicine and treatment. I had to put on my headphones and listen to Diana Krall to avoid the self-indulged conversation. I just don't want to hear it. Not that I am not compassionate about the issues, I just don't want to focus on them.

I am interested in focusing on getting through the challenges, and working on being healthy and normal.

> *"Health, happiness and success depend upon the fighting spirit of each person. The big thing is not what happens to us in life — but what we do about what happens to us."*
> *- George H. Allen*

I want to talk about what I can do in spite of how I feel, not what is difficult and doesn't feel good. I want to think about winning, not the consumption of illness. I may die, but so what, I'll make it right before I do and until I do! By the way, my plan is to live years.

I want to win not suffer. I will live in light, and not succumb to dark thoughts or behavior. I will live - to live, contribute and be positive.

Next treatment I am going to punch people in the side of the head to wake 'em up . . . OK, maybe not, But I will have my headphones on.

Friday, November 19, 2010 - Don't count the Chickens before the Eggs

While I am obviously not a doctor, and still need to have them render the opinion, I nevertheless just brought both PET scan studies home with

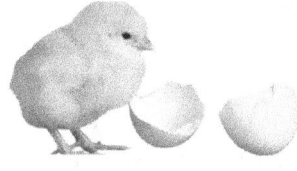

me after having a PET scan early this morning. For clarity, that would be the one I just had, and the one from September 23$^{rd to}$ compare it to.

To me, it appears that my rectal cancer is much smaller (maybe half), and it appears that the cancer in my lungs is disappearing. It is still there, but less of it, and some places it appears gone.

Again, I am not trained, but that is what it looks like to me. Officially I won't know until Monday.

I don't want to count the chickens before the eggs hatch but - I think I am headed down the right path.

A Personal Revelation
and Character Victory

Health wise, things had been rough up to this point, but it was because of the difficult journey, that two of life's most valuable lessons emerged.

1) The Lord Jesus added a commandment, to love one another. Little did I know how serious people had delivered on his word and

2) I found that it was vital for me to start understanding the word of God.

From this point forward in my journey, I became more intensely aware of the differences in what was really important versus the noise of my illness.

Monday, November 22, 2010 - Life's Lessons

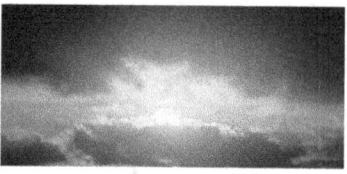

You may or may not believe in pre-ordained life or thinking. Who knows for sure? Maybe it is a combination. Maybe there are some broad stokes set in stone for your life, but I believe in free will. I think we can ignore or effect destiny.

For me, I have learned some important things in the last three months, which should have been on my radar screen long before now.

I have learned that I am so lucky to have the vast amount of people I have had pouring out their boundless love and support. It is the stuff feel good movies are made from, and I am grateful beyond measure.

It has opened my eyes and heart to realize and see something in human kind I never looked for prior to now.

Maybe I was arrogant, maybe just blind - whatever the reason, I wasn't seeing something in front of my face.

Not that it wasn't there all along; I just wasn't seeing the boundless generosity of humanity. I wouldn't recommend cancer as a way to expand your character, but it appears there can be a valuable lesson behind any experience. I am not happy about the illness, I am eternally grateful for the lesson.

Thanks to all of you, your generosity and God's grace - for now, I will live to share the value of this experience.

I am about 1/3 of the way through this skirmish, and am wondering if there are more surprise lessons waiting to conk me on the head.

Chapter 4 - Focus on Living

"Live as if your were to die tomorrow. Learn as if you were to live forever."   *-Gandhi*

By Thanksgiving of 2010, the health issues had begun to strip away much of the veneer that I had built into especially my work personality, exposing me to what really matters. That would be God, and the love shown to me by humanities' obedience to our Lord's commandment to love one another. I was really amazed and feeling that from many. It really shaped how I felt about the whole cancer experience.

I was no longer thinking about cancer's impact as the center piece of my life as much as how amazing it was to witness the abundant care, kindness and love that so many expressed almost daily.

That gave me a sense of responsibility to beat the disease, as I felt so many cheering me on to win the battle. Of course I felt this from family, but it extended far beyond that to include the medical staff like the infusion nurses, Alice, Brenda, Kathy, and Kim. Dr. Sam Shelanski made it clear that he cares. Friends, and colleagues from all over the world sent love in one way or another. People I don't even know began to follow the Blog.

All of the random acts of kindness and constant concern and love were like a powerful army standing with me to wage war. I may have been the only person suffering blows physically, but my army suffered blows emotionally in locked-step as the war progressed. I felt responsible for how all of us got through. This provided a powerful focus on positive thinking and energy. With so many invested in the battle, as the leader of the charge, I had to be positive. Souls depended on it, and cheered every success as if it were part of their own.

Cancer is not just about you. There is a wide circle of people that are impacted in varying degrees. Focus on helping them brings immeasurable rewards to you in joy and blessings of all sorts. You have to be strong on the inside, because physically you will be taking hard blows.

Thursday, November 25, 2010 - *Happy Thanksgiving*

Nothing like a brush with death to underscore what is important to living!

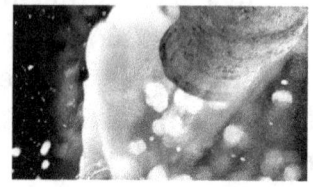

To me, of all the places I have been, or the things I have done, the most memorable, valuable, and treasured memories, always have to do with people.

Now it is Thanksgiving, and once again I am reminded of the most important and valuable parts of life, those we love and that love us. That bond is the irreplaceable treasure of life.

So, as I give thanks this year for God's abundance, I will open the Champaign and toast the people we love, and the irreplaceable treasure they add to life.

Here's to you . . . may you live long, love, and be loved.

Tuesday, November 30, 2010 – Round 5

*Tomorrow is round 5 of chemo.
One step away from being half
way through treatment. I am so
lucky that I already know that*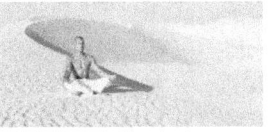
*the chemo is working, and that the outcome is good.
It makes dealing with the poisoning so much more
tolerable.*

*My long time friend Sue Klahr called Monday. She
beat cancer, from what appeared to be a difficult set
of circumstances. It was so helpful to talk with
someone that has been down the path. She
understood where I am, and knew, before me, where
I am going. Her perspective was immensely helpful.*

*Out of dark humor, we had a heartfelt belly laugh
when she told me she could tolerate the cancer, but
thought the chemo would kill her. Probably strange
to you, to think that is funny, but it is tickling the
"I've been there done that" funny bone.*

*Chemo is lousy, recovering and living is wonderful.
She pointed out, and I now agree, with why they call
people survivors. It is not easy, and it actually is an
accomplishment to make it through with mind, body
and soul - feeling healthy and hopeful.*

*My sincere wish for all of you is abundant health for
you and all you know. Cheers!*

Wednesday, December 1, 2010 - More Good News - The Gift of Life

My Chemo session always starts with a chat with my expert oncologist - Sam (MD). Today Sam started by telling 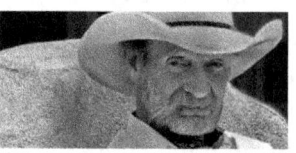 *Bonnie and I that the plan is changing. Instead of 12 total chemo treatments, it is being reduced to 8. In fact, at first chemo was through April, now it ends January 12th. So I am more than half way through - now!*

In the beginning, Sam told us I could have as little as a year. Now he says I am likely "long-term", which in his view means for my age the only acceptable outcome, is greater than 5 years, and he told us he is committed to do whatever it takes to make it happen.

I will still likely have a minor surgery to get rid of all traces of the colon cancer, but that is not a big deal. The strategy is that with the metastatic seed gone, and the wandering cancer cells dead from chemo, that I will live a long life. I like that plan, and am hopeful for that outcome.

So, now comes the "why me" question? **Answer;** *I don't know, and it doesn't matter. I can tell you, this has been a scary experience that has made me more ill than I have ever been. But, it has given me an abundant gratitude for the endless*

> *"Life's meaning can't be known by customary thought patterns, but by experience".*
>
> *- Albert Einstein*

bounty of loving, caring, and good people that cared for me in ways I didn't know they could, nor did I previously understand, or recognize. Most of all, Bonnie has really stood up for me and taken kind care of me.

The point: maybe God just wanted me to get the wake up call. What was the call? 1) It's a big beautiful world with you in it; 2) There are valuable lessons to any challenge and; 3) It is better to focus on the value, than the despair that can rob you of achieving knowledge that creates a positive outcome for you and all you know.

I consider the cancer challenge as that. It is a gift from God to grow, share, and someday comfort others, as you have for me.

I would add that you need to pay it forward, be grateful to have both the experience God provides, and the knowledge to share it in ways that bring value to others, as they need it.

In that way, I have benefited from all of you.

My humble thanks.

God's Message

It was around this time that I knew my mission was to write this book at some point. I heard the calling in the wee hours one morning, and tucked it away. I knew the cancer journey was a long one, and there were many twists and bumps ahead as God continued to drive the bus. As I am writing this, I have just completed my third bout with cancer and am in remission again, so I have seen and experienced a lot of things. I also know that my time may not be long, and that I need to get this done. I made a commitment that I would read the Bible cover to cover before I would write this book, because I felt it was important that if God was calling me to do this work that I had a reasonable grasp of God's work.

I started reading in February of 2012, and found I needed more help. I bought two different study Bibles and read them both, as well as listening to numerous sermons from a man I have not met but nevertheless love, Pastor and Doctor John McArthur who hails from Grace community church in Sun Valley, CA. Pastor McArthur authored one of the study Bibles. I am also attending church locally at Trinity Lutheran and really admire Pastor Ed Smith.

With all of that under my belt, I am under way!

But as you will see, the battle rages, but the blessings abound. Back to the blog. . .

Friday, December 3, 2010 - No Escape from Chemo

Ended round 5 of chemo today. They gave me an extra IV of saline to try to keep me from getting ill. No good, I'm ill. You just can't dose up on poison and escape the symptoms.

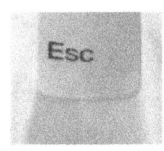

I have a bifurcated brain, one half is jumping for joy knowing I am winning and will recover, the other half is just tired of being tired and ill with chemo.

That's just medicine. You may not like it, but that is the path back to health. I am grateful to be on the mend, but the path to recovery I could do without. But then, if I skipped that, those great lessons from life may not have happened. Strange eh?

I will get through this, and I am anxious for it to end.

39 days to go. Please keep sending the healing vibes and prayers.

Monday, December 6, 2010 – On the Up-Swing

Well I made it through chemo weekend.

I worked on a very complex spreadsheet all day to calculate storage requirements for video capture, with a multitude of variables, like compression rates, frame rates, frames size, hours, and cameras. Which should tell you that I am able to think and work. I'm certainly not fully up, but I am better today than yesterday, and tomorrow will be better than today.

So, I am headed back up to the top of the roller coaster, and then on December 15th, I will barrel back down.

Only 3 more times! Whoopee!

Friday, December 10, 2010 - High Five to the Real Heroes!!

I don't know about you, but I had a fast a furious week. It is interesting that a person can sometimes do more than you would otherwise expect. For me, I came off of a chemo weekend, 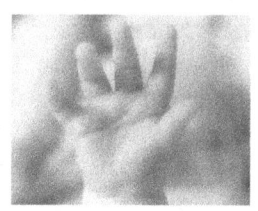 *Monday arrived, work started, I had a ton of stuff to get done, and through the week - did!*

I find it interesting how different people handle difficult and challenging situations.

I like the way Henry Ward Beecher put it: "Troubles are often the tools by which God fashions us for better things."

For me, in addition to a seemingly huge amount of poison pumped into me twice a month, I have also received some valuable and humbling insights. Among other things, empathy comes to mind.

Prior to getting cancer, hearing about somebody with cancer affected me through a type of conscience immunity. To really appreciate cancer, is just one of those things that require you to walk in someone's moccasins to get, at least it was for me. Now that I am wearing those moccasins, I have recently been knocked in the head with an empathy bat.

Now when I hear yet another story of somebody's cancer plight, I have a much deeper and realistic understanding of the challenge. Last weekend I heard about an NFL offensive coach that had chemo

the previous day, and was calling plays the next day
at the big game. Holly cow! I have to tell you the
day after chemo there is a real phenomenon, in the
inner circles it is known as "chemo brain". Its real
and it is a fog to look out from.

You know, there are a lot of pretty amazing people
out there that carry on life in-spite of their
challenges.

I have to tell you, while my challenge hasn't been
easy, the challenge that many face dwarfs what has
been thrown at me so far. I'm doing fine for the
circumstances.

Other people with far greater issues are walking
torches, lighting a path that few have taken or ever
will, even though the daily rigors they face would
floor most anyone you know.

With all of that to carry around, they happily offer
inspiration to many they know, and often to many
they don't know, or ever will. They don't care and it
doesn't matter. They have a vision to share that aids
those that have a need, they send it out, and people
benefit. It is the sole purpose, there is no gain, there
is only loving care.

Then there are those that have given and have made
a huge contribution to the circles of people their lives
have touched. Some of them eventually succumb to
the eventual wrath of the unending progress of the
disease. Many of them seem to have fought bravely,
inspired brilliantly, and in the end are just worn
down and out. They are told the end of the road is

near, and they seem to rapidly, just know how to gracefully return to God.

Talk about an exit strategy. I see it as graduation day.

By the way, I am nowhere close to any of that, but I can now see it, really understand it, and have a reverend appreciation and respect for those that with so little to spare, have offered so much more than those with what appears to be everything, including health.

I've noticed that heroes and ignorance are never self-aware.

Heroes don't need a message, the ignorant need an empathy bat.

Cancer is a Thief

While on chemo, there are many life events that you miss. One of the problems with chemo is that it can shut down your immunization system. That makes getting and infection, or flu, or a cold - potentially very dangerous. So going to your nephew's birthday party, or attending a holiday meal with the family is off limits.

Another issue is that you are robbed of strength and stamina. As such, there are things you want to do that you simply cannot.

Tuesday, December 14, 2010 - Disappointment Maximized

Tomorrow will be round 6 of 8.

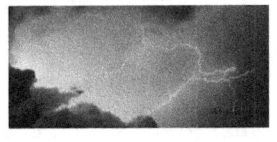

I'm trying to preserve my life; my friend Fred Moore just lost his wife Molly.

I am crushed by this news. I scarcely know what to think. It reminds me of how precious and at the same time how precarious life is. Today may be the last chance you get to do what is right, to settle something or to let someone you know how much you care.

Molly's memorial service is this Friday at 2pm. My Chemo begins tomorrow, and runs through Friday at noon. There isn't a person on this planet I respect or look up to more than Fred Moore. In addition to family and personal friends, the people that will attend Molly's service in support of our friend Fred, will be the cream of the IT industry. People that have worked with and have grown to love Fred, and his family.

For me, I am in deep struggle. I want to stand up for Fred and his family by being among the multitudes of family and friends that will be at the service. Yet, in my own health struggles, and just coming off of being injected with poison for 48 continuous hours, I doubt that I can physically manage being there, and I am just crushed at the thought of not being there to support my friend Fred.

I think of every thing that has happened along the way in my personal battle, this is the most disturbing. I want to go to pay my respect for a man at the top of the list of people I respect, and probably can't.

It just breaks my heart.

Thursday, December 16, 2010 - Are you enjoying your Chemo today?

Chemo is cumulative. The longer you are on it, the lousier it becomes. Think of a ball dropped from shoulder height. The first 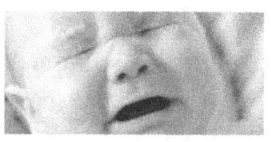 *bounce is relatively high compared to the next. The next bounce is less and so on. Recovery cycles are like that. Early on it was no big deal and the symptoms weren't so bad. It is getting worse.*

By the time I saw my oncologist (Sam) this time, he understood how difficult it is becoming, and decided to push my next treatment out another week to give my body a chance to recover. That's a big relief for me!

Which means the next treatment is 1/5/11 now. I will get through Christmas probably feeling pretty decent.

The really great news is that I only have two more to go after this treatment and it is over. Friday I will sink, Saturday I will hit bottom, Sunday I will be up and moving around, Monday I will be able to work. But it isn't easy.

It isn't the cancer that is making me feel so lousy, it's the treatment. Bittersweet stuff. I am happy to take the meds cause I have a lot to live for. But it's like going in to get a really lousy flu. It is just hard to do.

I'm just complaining here folks. Have to keep this in perspective; I am going to be just fine, and soon. *The final steps are the hardest in this case. But by February I will be well on my way back to full health. Just have to hang tough a bit longer.*

When I wrote this, I was under the impression that if I could make cancer go away it was over.

Later, another oncologist used the metaphor, "the horses are out of the barn." Meaning - cancer is running around my body, and it will be back.

At present, I have been through five bouts of cancer. I now expect cancer to return, and I further expect it will eventually kill me.

Two more to go. Better days ahead.

Thank God for the miracle healing. Despise Satan for the Chemo, which was undoubtedly invented by one of his clan. Just kidding - my wicked humor at play again.

Monday, December 20, 2010 - Merry Christmas Everybody!

Well I made it through chemo weekend! My body was beaten up, however my spirits are high, and I 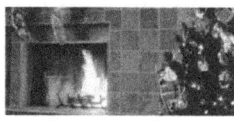 *am better today! I can now look forward to having an extra week off chemo, which should help me to recover from all of the poison. That is really great because David (son) and Kim (daughter in-law) are driving up, and Marci (daughter) will be here too.*

An old fashion Chalfant Christmas with everyone here. Awesome!

Bonnie and I hope all of you have the best Christmas ever, and a terrific 2011 as well.

For my Jewish friends, Happy Hanukkah, which I now know isn't exactly the same, but a friend and I recently had a lively conversation, which helped to spread some light on me.

Monday, December 27, 2010 – Look Up, Priorities

Recently the West Coast, and in particular Southern California has been hammered with rain. Lots of rain, and in a short period of time. California always seems to have problems. Last summer it was fire, now its rain. With vegetation burned and gone, now there are floods of mud.

Last week, I watched a highly distressed woman, shown near her house that was filled with 4 feet of mud. She and her children escaped from a second floor window with an emergency ladder. During the news interview, the lady was hysterically screaming, "I HAVE NOTHING, I HAVE NOTHING!!!!"

So here I am thinking, maybe she would have felt better if she had lost her daughter but still had her new couch and her big screen TV.

Look, I like things as much as the next person, especially techno stuff. But lately it occurs to me that when I show up at the pearly gates I doubt that I will be judged by what I have accumulated, or any other material measure. I think the measurement will be more about what I gave, not what I got.

The funny thing about the hysterical woman is that she is probably more typical than atypical. The sad part is, why does it take a brush with death to realize what the important parts of life are?

I guess it doesn't for everybody, but there is no doubt that that is what it took for me. How many knot-heads like me are out there? Probably more than I realize, similar to my recent discovery that the big value measurement isn't love of life, but life of love.

What did you give today? What difference did you make? Did you notice the selfless act of someone you know? I have seen a lot of that lately. Not that it wasn't always going on around me; it's just that I now have open eyes.

I'm embarrassed to feel like I am on the pulpit, but I feel like I have stumbled upon the most important lesson of my life. Perhaps it is the most important lesson of life.

I have always admired those that can learn from the experiences of others, all of us know the multitudes of people that sadly cannot. The frustration of that alone, makes me want to express my appreciation for my new and deeper understanding of life's values and the greatness that exists in the hearts of humanity.

Maybe it is for that very reason, that God's messenger to greater truth, is delivered through the challenge of adversity. Who knows what good things wait for the hysterical lady if she were to simply choose to climb the mountain? On the other hand, how desperate can her situation become if she cannot see or follow the opportunities that are presented, as the fall of one chapter closes and the spring of another takes root.

It is up to her, you and I can decide what value comes from each challenge. I believe in looking up, not down.

What do you believe?

Tuesday, January 4, 2011 - Getting Close to Conclusion

It's been almost three weeks since I was last poisoned and I feel great! Gee what a surprise, stop getting poisoned, feel great. Who knew?

I have to admit, it will be difficult in some ways to go in tomorrow, knowing I will be getting poisoned and not feeling well for days. That's the price of health however, so it is OK. I am getting really excited about having this behind me. I am so looking forward to getting on with life, and moving past having cancer run my life.

I am still grateful for all of the lessons, and for expanding my vision. But I am not going to focus on that at the moment.

I just wanted to update my status to let you good folks know that all is well, and I am almost through!

Hip, hip, HOORAY!

Thursday, January 6, 2011 – Chemo – Heaven or Hell? A day in the life of Chemo

Saw my oncologist Sam yesterday. Bottom line is that he fully expects to see me in remission when I get the next PET (Positron Emission Tomography) scan later this month, which occurs after the next and final chemo session. Of course there are no guarantees, and only the PET scan will objectively measure reality. But Sam is experienced, smart, and optimistic based on everything he is looking at including on-going blood analysis.

If anything is left, the Chemo will likely be dropped, and only the Avastin treatment will continue, which without the chemo will leave me symptom free. That could go on for a short while. On the other hand, if the rectal cancer is reduced sufficiently, then the next step would be to wait six to eight weeks to get the Avastin out of my system, and then a minor surgery to remove the evil seed (tumor).

The reason I would have to wait is that the Avastin is known to cause uncontrollable hemorrhaging, which of course is fatal. By the way, all of that plus the current mondo headaches, high blood pressure and hyper acidy in my stomach – sheeze!

However, what a contrast from the beginning of all of this skirmish. In the beginning the news continued to get worse regularly, with an outcome that resulted in death. That causes some unique thinking - let me tell you.

Through the grace of God, friendly genetics, unfettered love, support, prayers, and care - every visit is now upbeat and looking better. It appears now that I will beat stage four cancer and live indefinitely. My worst fear now is getting run over by a beer truck.

I thank God and all of you for winning.

So that's the good news.

The bad news is that nothing has changed with treatment, and chemo is still lousy. I was infused from 9:30am yesterday until 2pm. Sure enough the poison has made me ill and stupid. I am wearing a pump now, and through Friday morning - that will continue to infuse me with a chemo agent called Fluorouracil or 5FU for short. It is one of three agents I take, collectively in the oncology world they are known as "Full Fury." From my point of view, that is an appropriate name.

So, on a positive note the treatment is working for which I am grateful, with the downside of being back down in the bottom of the well and feeling chemo ill. I had three weeks off and was feeling better than I have since August, until getting chemo-charged, yuck.

Even so, I will finish a complex technical assessment today of a client infrastructure, and write a proposal for an analyst sponsored WebEx on virtualization strategy and benefits when using either an array or stack management schema. That will have me focused on what I love, not how I feel.

Thanks for reading my blog and for your generous support that has been a major and serious contribution to healing.

May God bless all of you, by keeping you and all you love safe and healthy.

Monday, January 10, 2011 – Quack - Still here

As expected the weekend was what I call a chemo weekend. I wasn't feeling so well, so I watched too much football. I also got a few things done, but a lot of rest. I mostly concentrated on learning how to administer my new OS X server.

Feeling pretty good today as I climb back out of the chemo hole. I have lots of meetings and stuff to do today. The first con call starts at 0700. Bring 'em on.

We are having a snow day.

Hope all of you are well!

Saturday, January 15, 2011 – Looking Forward To Better Days!

Cancer is like a grenade, it has a powerful impact on the person who finds out they have it, and there is 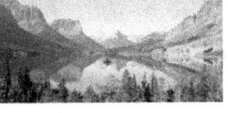 *the potential of a lot of collateral damage in expanding circles around you.*

You never know how any human will react to the news, either as the person who has cancer, or on how your circle of family and friends will react.

I have found that whether it is family or friends, there are some people that jump into your life to offer spiritual, love, physical, emotional, and any other kind of support you can think of, as well as some you probably wouldn't expect. And then there are people, either through lack of interest, or demons they don't know how to face, that retract and you never hear from.

On balance, I would say the latter seems to be a minor percentage. It actually makes me want to comfort them, which I have in some cases. In other cases some people haven't or won't return my call. Must be scary for them, I don't know. I do know some people have just said they don't know what to say. Personally, I think I have learned that what is said isn't important, telling somebody you care is.

It has been a profound experience to hear from so many people I care about, and hear stories of how I have had an impact on their lives.

The blessing is that I didn't have to wait until I die to hear it in the form of a eulogy.

I was fortunate enough to hear it while I am alive. It may be a bit like the role that Jimmy Stewart played in the movie "It's a Wonderful Life". In his role, George Bailey had the opportunity to find out there was a complicated trail of positive impact that his presence had made to a large circle of family and friends.

While I have no idea what the world would look like without my existence, I can tell you that I have been deeply moved by the amount of people that have expressed various experiences we have shared together, and what the impact was to them. I can also tell you, it will bring tears to your eyes, if you are ever fortunate enough to experience what I have.

No money can buy that, for a fortunate few, it comes for free when circumstance are right. It has changed many views I have on life, and I am so grateful for that, and for all of you that contributed to an awakening within the spirit of the composition of who I am and who I have become.

So three cheers to you, and a Colorado Mountain of gratitude.

I have one more chemo session to get through. The last one was difficult, I expect the next one will be as well physically; however, emotionally and intellectually, I am reeling with excitement mixed with a dose of caution.

Sam, my Oncologist, expects to find me in remission after the next PET scan near the end of this month.

If that turns out to be the case, by early February, I expect to be feeling great again. I will still have a minor surgery to remove what I call the "evil seed" six to eight weeks after the last chemo, but from where I sit that looks like an insignificant speed bump.

So here's to better days!

I am optimistically looking forward to health, and looking to find a way to help anyone I can to find his or her way to an easier path through a difficult journey, just as you have helped me.

Tuesday, January 18, 2011 – 7 Down, 1 to Go!

Tomorrow will be the final chemo treatment, so long cancer - hello life! I will know the exact status of the 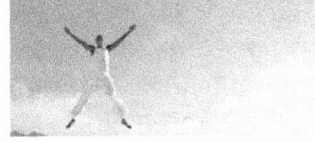 *cancer after the next PET scan, which will be in a couple of weeks.*

In the meanwhile - I am elated to be at the end of the poisoning, and dreading the final installment at the same time.

So - about two more weeks of feeling like a zombie, and then I will finally climb out of this hole - hopefully forever.

I feel like I have beaten the grim reaper, I still have to pay taxes however. One out of two of the big ones - not bad.

I am also wondering if anyone will want the stuff they sent to me, back?

Oops - wicked humor again.

By the way, you wouldn't believe how gracious my company Nexsan, has been to me. They have been so supportive, understanding, and accommodating. Words like "thank you" are not adequate.

Monday, January 24, 2011 - The Waiting Game

In the beginning I was told I would die in about a year. That was before all of the determination I threw at the issue, and the prayers and loving support all of you threw at it.

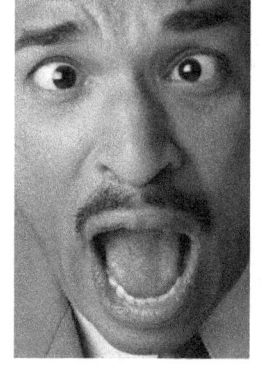

It appears that determination, prayers, love and support were stronger than the disease because I have now finished the last chemo treatment, and Sam, my Oncologist, fully expects me to be cancer free.

I have a PET scan in Fort Collins Monday the 31st, and will have the official results Feb 2nd. Of course, I will ask for the scan results before I leave the radiology office, so that I can come home and look at the modality myself, as I pretend to be a qualified radiologist, and preview the PET. I will also, of course, render and opinion, and let you know what Dr. Charlatan Chalfant thinks.

In the meanwhile, I felt terrible over the weekend, physically. However, emotionally I am overjoyed with optimism - believing I am better, and will not have to have any more treatments. Spiritually I am grateful to all of you and what I see as one of God's miracles.

But of course, all of that thinking is just me and the power of positive thinking. The reality is - I won't know with any medical certainty, until February 2nd.

Until then I have a new challenge. Now I get to wait, and wonder - as I recover from all of the poisoning I have been through as a stark reminder of what I would like to not repeat.

Next week will be a pivotal week in my life. By the time I get whatever the news will be, I should be feeling pretty good physically. I hope the news on the 2nd will be good emotionally.

Until then, I will wait, and try not to over-think it.

Tick-tock - I wonder what the Doc will say?

Monday, January 31, 2011 - Dr. Chalfant's View (a true Charlatan)

I had the positron emission tomography (PET) scan early this morning; the picture above is the PET machine I was in.

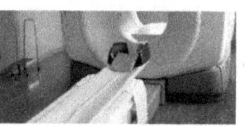

Bonnie and I looked at the results, and compared them to past scans for an hour or so today.

I can't conclude anything with certainty, but here are my unqualified perspectives:

- *The cancer in my lungs is gone*

- *The cancer in my colon is reduced by 50% again, just as it was the last time*

- *There are spots in other places I don't understand and to me are questionable*

The official and qualified results will happen Wednesday morning.

Wednesday, February 2, 2011 – I Win, Almost done . . .

Just spoke to Sam, my oncologist.

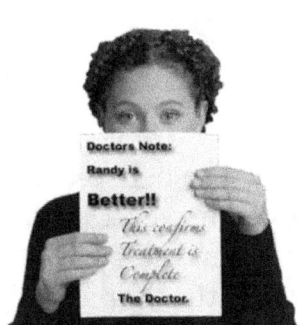

- *No more cancer in my Lungs*

- *No new cancer in my body*

- *Small amount left in my Rectum*

- *Surgery in 4 weeks to remove*

- *No radiation*

  - *No more Chemo*

I am going to live, and be fine.

The Grim Reality (The perspective from July 2012)

This news was great, but not accurate. There never was a surgery because doctors finally agreed it could not be done.

I also believed at the time that the game was over, however it was just the opening salvo. At present there have been two more cancer bouts since then for a total of three.

The cancer was never "gone"; it was just inactive for short periods. In reality, it is highly probable it will kill me eventually, and that I will just continue to have cancer, get treatment, it goes into remission for a while, then it comes back. Eventually my body stops responding to the chemo and I die. There is an outside chance that will take many years, but the probabilities are that it will happen within a few years.

Sunday, February 6, 2011 - Post Cancer Thinking

I think you have to walk the path to ultimately know what it is like to go through the discovery that you have cancer, and the rough road to 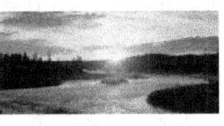 *healing. So I thought I would share my thoughts.*

For me when the medical team first said the word "cancer" in their explanation for what was going on with me, I had a physical reaction that was chest tightening. It just frightened me enough that I physically felt it go right through me.

Within a few minutes of the doctor leaving me, I just sort of released it into the hand of our Lord Jesus Christ, and thought destiny has its own course. Oddly, even then I didn't believe it would be a death sentence. Of course the initial view was that it was just a colon tumor.

The big blow was when Sam, my oncologist, ordered a stat lung biopsy. Just before Bonnie and I went over to the hospital, he informed us that if it was cancer in my lungs it was not curable, and that at best (statistically), I had not much more than a year to live. A few hours later, and after the biopsy, a doctor at the hospital confirmed it was indeed cancer. That physically gripped me too. But, again after a few minutes of thought, I still didn't believe it was a guaranteed death sentence, and that no matter what, I would face the music and do whatever was needed to be done, in order to heal.

So - I started the chemo regime. At first it wasn't difficult. Going forward, each treatment was more difficult than the last. By the end, it was a struggle to go through a treatment. However, midway through, I had a PET scan and knew that my body was responding favorably. That was the first good news we had, in months of progressively worse news. It was very encouraging and made it more tolerable to know that even though the treatment was difficult, I was headed in the right direction.

At the end of the treatment I found out the life threatening cancer in my lungs was gone. That also elicited a physical response from me, and it seems that the same happened to many of you when you heard the news as well.

I found that the incredible reaction by so many of you to the news that I had cancer made an unexpected and huge difference in helping my resolve to win.

I had a sense that not only could I not let my family down, I could not let all of the people that were sending prayers, love, and support down - as well. It gave me focus to ignore the physical issues of chemo, keep working, and trust God to carry me through. In fact, working was a blessing, because it allowed me to focus on what I love, not on how I felt.

I have found that the human outpouring of support in a multitude of different ways is a very humbling experience. I of course never experienced it before at this level, and I just can't adequately express how much it impacted me. For one thing it seems to have activated an emotional response that I have never really had. It seems to have made me hyper-aware of the joy of human accomplishment, as well as the impact of any human trauma.

I don't mean just as awareness, I seem to feel it now. It is like an exposed trigger. I don't know if it is a good thing or a bad thing. But it is real, I am empathetically hyper aware in ways I have never been before. As a technical type personality, perhaps I have not had an emotional balance for human challenges – I do now – in a big way.

More than anything else, I find that with all of this newfound empathy, and having a deeper understanding for the fears and challenges of a life threatening illness, that I would be very happy if I were able to help people that may be prone to allow the fear and suffering control how they feel. Of course there is fear and it is unquestionably physically difficult.

But those things <u>do not have to define who you are</u>. To me, your identity should not change.

It seems really important to have the strength of character to maintain a sense of priority for remembering who you are, what you care about, and staying positive about where the journey is leading you by trusting the care givers and divine providence. They know what they are doing. Let them worry about setting the course. That gives you the freedom to just try to do your best.

In the end, it seems that the more difficult the challenge, the more valuable the lesson.

I would never have chosen the challenge of cancer to add value to my character. By the same token, I honestly feel that it has added an irreplaceable awaking within me to human generosity, God's grace, and proof that even in the darkest and most desperate hours, faith and a steady commitment can bring victory, knowledge, and ultimately for me, a personality and spiritual awakening driving me to want to try to help others get through their difficult path.

At the moment, I don't know where that will lead. On the other hand, I believe that God will let me know if and when the time is right.

Until then, I still have one more step to get through, surgery. Somehow that feels like a speed bump compared to everything else. No big deal, but the end of a rough road. Thank God – literally.

Thanks to all of you too. Believe it or not, you made a difference. Now it's my turn to help.

Wednesday, February 23, 2011 – The Long and Winding Road

Nothing is easy that's worthwhile. That applies to health and getting past cancer.

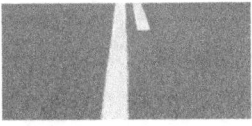

I just got back from seeing my Oncologist Sam. Here's the current view.

I am going to get scheduled in the next few days to have another ultrasound/colonoscopy. That will give us a current view of what is happening with the tumor/cancer.

From that, we will choose a course of action from one of three options:

1. *Tumor larger (I already know from the recent PET scan this isn't the case)*

    a. *Radiation and then Surgery*

2. *Tumor smaller, but still there (most likely)*

    a. *Surgery and then Chemo*

3. *Tumor gone (not too unlikely)*

    a. *Chemo (6 treatments over 12 weeks)*

The good news is I am no longer fighting death, which is what the cancer in my lungs was all about. The bad news is that, as Sam my Oncologist tells me, this is like a street fight. If it is option number 3 that makes sense, he not only wants to do chemo, he wants to do a more aggressive form of chemo to kick it while it is down.

Which means I will get beaten up again for three months - except it will be worse. On a positive note, he talked about two other cases that he has won with people that had metastasized colon cancer to the liver (more difficult than my case).

So, he is confident that he is going to cure me - which is great. But again, it looks likely that I will have to endure three more months of difficult chemo treatment.

Wednesday, March 16, 2011 – Chin-up, Not what I wanted

Well the results are in. The cancer in my colon has shrunk, but not all that much.

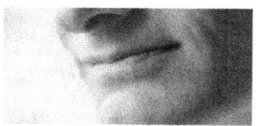

So the plan is as suspected, I start chemo next week again, which will last for three months - once every other week. At the end of that, we will re-evaluate. If it has shrunk enough by then, then we will do surgery. After that, if there is anything left - more chemo or maybe radiation. Who knows. . .

The good news is that I am no longer fighting for my life. The bad news is that I have to take chemo again. That's the cost of health, so that is what I will do, but I am not looking forward to it.

Sunday, March 27, 2011 - Light at the end of the Tunnel

The news I received on Wednesday when I saw my oncologist Sam, was better than expected. It turns out that the original size of the tumor was 14 cubic centimeters, throughout all of the previous chemo; it has shrunk down to 4 cubic centimeters, or a reduction of 71.43%. That happened through a course of 8 treatments of chemo, one every other week. So that's good.

The trick now is to get the remaining cancer in my colon to go away. I had my first round of this regimen of chemo Wednesday of last week. One down, 5 to go. It seems reasonable to believe that I can shrink the rest down to nothing in the next 5 treatments ending June 1st. The next PET scan will tell the story. That will happen in June as well.

In the meanwhile, I have 5 more treatments to get through. Things are going about as expected. Get poisoned, feel terrible, and get better.

I feel pretty decent today. But I also know it will get worse as I go along. Even so, the cancer in my lungs is gone, and I am going to live. The remaining cancer in my rectum, is going away. There is light at the end of the tunnel, and I will be fine in time.

It seems that more than anything, this is now a test of patience and that is a difficult challenge for me. I can't imagine anyone that wouldn't get tired of being ill. Yet, I have seen so many cancer patients that have had a far worse ride than me. I may be battling cancer, but I am so lucky compared to many, and for that I am grateful.

I am also awed by Bonnie's patience. She seems to be quite happy to go about serving me meals and looking after my comfort. I get annoyed with myself for feeling ill, it's amazing that she seems to stay happy regardless. I think she is better and kinder than I am, something for me to aspire to.

Tuesday, April 5, 2011 - Chemo - I'm Laughing at you!

There are as many ways to deal with and look at cancer, as there are people that have it. As you know, I have managed to stay pretty positive and strong. Don't get me wrong, I'm still OK, but chronic illness is getting on my nerves.

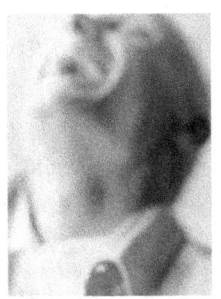

I can't afford to just let go of my emotions, and somehow come unglued. But I am also annoyed enough with all of this that it would be easy to go sour. That of course is not going to happen, but I am close enough to the issue that I can see it.

Just realize that I know that the cancer that made it to my lungs was going to kill me, and I am now past that. What's left is MUCH easier to resolve, with every indication that I will beat this. All of that is oh-so-logical.

Emotionally, I have had thoughts like - "will I ever be healthy again?" I hear that thought going through my head, and automatically slam on the brakes.

Self-doubt is not productive, and I insist on control over that. But isn't it interesting that even with a rational view, and knowing that the outcome is looking good that I can still have doubts creeping around my head waiting to grab on.

I think it is probably all very normal under the circumstances. And maybe my normal is different than anyone else. But it is still easy to see that large doses of poison followed by being very ill, can upset reasonable thinking.

No matter what, rest assured knowing that I will keep up the battle and positive attitude about all of this. Last week a friend mentioned that I now know what a rat feels like after dining on poison. That tickled, if not inspired a surge in my wicked humor.

So Chemo - I'm laughing at you! You may poison me, you can make me ill, but my spirit remains intact, and I refuse to succumb to the assault. I won't be robbed. I have a mission to complete; I'll be around to complete that.

Thanks to all of you that continue to offer your support and prayers. Unless you have been in a similar spot, you may not know how much it matters.

Wednesday, April 20, 2011 - Wyatt Earp was never shot

Well the last two weeks has been a bit bumpy. I find that with the new chemo, I seem to be OK to work during the day, but that is all the energy I have. Once that energy is burned up, I plummet. Weekends are just rest and recovery.

As you probably know, chemo also lowers ones immunization system. The more harsh form of chemo I am now taking also lowered mine. That resulted in getting a staph infection, which got the medical types I see excited. It turns out that the staph I have is not the variety known as Methicillin-Resistant Staphylococcus Aureus (MRSA) so it won't kill me. I was on top of it, so it also didn't get away from me. It is resolving slowly but surely.

In the meanwhile, I went in for my chemo, and they bounced me this week for fear that the additional reduction in my immune system would allow the staph to further develop, which could be life threatening. So I skipped a week. Not so bad, except that means my completion date is now a week longer too. Seems strange that anyone would care I suppose. It's just that this is nasty stuff, and I want it to end sooner than later.

Work wise, I have a large amount of projects I am working, and thank God, because it is fun. I am doing a lot of writing at the moment and enjoying it so much. I am focused on writing solutions briefs, and have many in my work queue to complete. I have completed two in the last two weeks, and feel really good about how they came out. That's the stuff that I really like doing. Its nice that I have the focus to do them, and that they need to be done! By the way, that's about 65% of my time, the rest is doing all of the other things that pop up or must be done. Nexsan is great. The most enjoyable job I have had in years.

Anyway, I have about 50 more days of this skirmish to deal with, and hopefully everything will turn out OK at the end of that. It sure looks like it so far! Keep your fingers crossed!

Friday, April 29, 2011 – New Plan

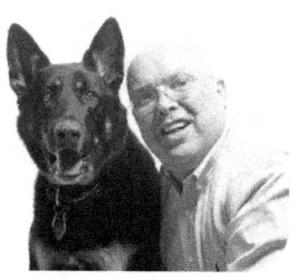

Roxy, my baby

It became obvious to the Oncologists that I am getting beaten up pretty well. The chemo I am on is rough, then a staph infection, and other issues. Bonnie and I saw Sam on Wednesday. I think we have a negotiated truce.

The new plan is that I have one more chemo session, then a PET scan. OK, here comes the Boolean logic, if the cancer is still there, more chemo, else it is gone, in which case I go in for yet another Colonoscopy. While having the colonoscopy, they may decide to do a resection (cut a chunk out) or scrape, or do nothing. They won't know until they see what they have.

But if I am lucky, I may get to avoid more chemo after the next round. I am leaving the status on the top "How's Randy" Blog page showing all the treatments, and the clock running to the end, so I don't get too excited.

I just got off the chemo pump today and expect to be down this weekend. So more Rest & Relation to steel up for next week.

One more session of chemo, and maybe I get lucky. Cross whatever you can for me! No matter what, this is winding down. The final leg of the journey is the most difficult, but that is expected with chemo. I am still holding up, and will make it through. I just hope I catch a break and finish a little early.

Hey - have I told all of you I love you lately? Well I do, thanks for hanging in there with me!

Friday, May 13, 2011 – One more PET Scan

Well I just finished this round of chemo. I don't have another round officially scheduled, even though there could be more.

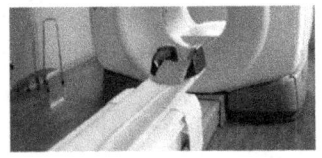

Next stop is the PET scan, which will happen the morning of the 24th. I have a meeting with Sam on the 25th to get the results. The hope is that the cancer is gone and I am finished with chemo. Sam thinks I have something like a 50-70% probability of it being gone.

So I am just hanging in there - trying to get over the effects of poison, and hoping this challenge is winding down or better yet over. I have a taste for life, and am anxious to get back to living it normally.

I have posted much in this blog on my outlook, gratitude, and philosophy. None of that has lessened - it only deepens. Since I think I have covered it well, I am not going to do more of it now except for one point.

I was talking to a guy at the infusion center today. His problems are gigantic compared to mine, to which he said, he was grateful, because there is always someone who is worse. He said it twice in a row while waving a hand dismissively. It floored me. I feel that way, and so does he from a far more bleak position.

The human spirit is generous beyond my previous understanding, and the human spirit is courageous beyond my current understanding.

God has to be watching and admiring these people with such huge challenges, hearts and gracious minds.

Wednesday, May 25, 2011 - Battle won for now

Well the battle is over. I am in complete remission.

I haven't had time to properly reflect on this yet, as I just received the news. However, I am flooded with thoughts.

It will take a couple of days to assimilate my thoughts, conclusions, and understanding of the blessings I have received.

I am overwhelmed by the news to be sure, and will share the post battle thinking soon.

Love and gratitude to all of you.

Saturday, May 28, 2011 – The Aftermath

I don't think anybody grows up thinking they will have cancer. Did you? Nobody has cancer until the day things aren't right, 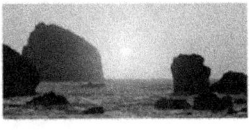 *you go to a doctor to find out why, and you wind up getting the news.*

When I was told I have cancer I physically felt my whole body instantly tighten from stress and fear. The news is frightening, the future and the possibility of a future are suddenly uncertain.

We have all heard stories of horrible experiences people endure through cancer treatments, including radiation, chemo, and surgeries. Who in their right mind would want that? Nobody I know of, and certainly not me.

Sometimes life doesn't offer a good choice. Even though you may not like the choices available, there are always choices. For me the choice was do nothing and die, or do the program and hope to live.

So why do that? Personally I am looking forward to the day I die. If you believe in God, heaven, and the hereafter, why would you not want that? From my perspective that beats anything I can have here on Earth. But its not always what any individual wants. I feel obligated to live, to provide for my family that depends on me, to be a husband, to be a dad, to take care of my disabled daughter, to take care of my dogs, to live up to the commitments I have made to a circle of family, friends, and colleagues.

I didn't feel like I had an option, I am committed to many responsibilities, and therefore there was only one choice, live, get through treatments, and beat cancer.

Cancer treatment is difficult; it makes you sick, and tired, more than you have probably ever known. Yet, living through cancer treatment doesn't have to be about how sick and tired you are. Oh - it will limit you, and it also limits and impacts people around you. But it doesn't have to define <u>who you are</u>, <u>or will be</u>.

It is simply a large challenge. Maybe it is like trying to climb Mt. Everest. Have you done that? Do you have any idea how difficult it is? How dangerous it is? How much suffering you would have to endure? So why do people do that? Certainly not for the danger, pain and suffering. They do it to feel the exhilaration of the victory over a difficult challenge that few on this planet can claim.

Well friends, the battle with cancer can be very similar. The defining characteristic of winning the battle is about keeping your eye on the <u>prize</u>, not the pain and suffering, or the danger.

The "prize" is patiently waiting for the doctors' visit when you learn you are in remission and have won the most difficult, scary, and challenging objective in your life.

Cancer survivors have climbed the mountain, and have planted a flag at the top that says - "I won." They have survived physical and emotional challenges that are as difficult, craggy, and dangerous as any human endeavor has ever been. Not that there aren't other human illness or challenges that aren't equal or greater, because there are. But Cancer is a big one, and nobody knows how big until you and people around you are there.

It is a far better and rewarding path to get through cancer by aligning yourself with the win.

I have won for now. It could come back, but to me it is the same as getting off the mountain. I have planted the flag, now I have to survive getting back down. The journey is not over until I am safely back to base camp and healthy. It is still dangerous; there can be slips and storms I don't know about yet. But just like the commitment to summit, I am now committed to getting home safely. I will be here to live up to commitments to family, friends, and colleagues.

You may not appreciate the tremendous influence you may have on the will of another to survive. But believe me, it is a major positive force. I have been incredibly touched by the love, care and support that I have been flooded with. There is no possible way to repay that debt, so I will simply say thank you. You made a difference.

Someday I will meet our maker, but not today. Today I will take action to continue to improve, get stronger, stay vigilant, and continue the journey.

So here's to victory and life, and the people we love. May all of you win your battles, overcome challenges, plant your flags, and return home safely.

More to Come

The end of May was a joyful time. I had won the battle. Little did I realize that it was a short-lived victory. Just over 4 months later cancer had returned. Even so, my faith in God kept me calm and peaceful.

Wednesday, October 5, 2011 - The Gift that Keeps on Giving

This entry is going to be short and to the point.

I went for my first post cancer checkup, and had a PET scan. The news is that cancer is back, and it's moderately aggressive. I have one rather large and active spot in my right lung, and the rectal cancer is active again as well. There about 11 other places in my lungs that are involved.

So this is serious, statistically I have from one to three years to live. The big fear is that it metastasizes to my liver. That could make things take a bad turn.

I begin chemo on the 26th of this month, and will be on it until early February on the current plan. There is also a possibility that I will be doing some clinical trial drugs.

OK, that was the brutal truth - so that is out of the way.

I don't believe that most of you read this blog for that, I think you like the philosophical view of things that stem from the brutal truth. If that is true for you, I have some really good news!

I have been spending lots of time trying to figure out God, the Universe, and the meaning of life. While I don't have many answers to any of that, I do have lots of thought, good and bad, up and down; I have also developed many questions.

I am actually looking forward to writing. It helps me to settle some of the questions, and organize thinking. It is especially rewarding that many of you have been so positive about following the story as it develops, and hearing back from you regarding the positives you get from it.

So if you're inclined - tune-in, and we will explore the developments, the discoveries of what some of us think is really important, versus the noise and distraction, and maybe - I will get to share the joy of a miracle. If not, I will share the expectations I have of meeting our maker.

I have to tell you, I am strangely calm, and resolved. While I am not happy with what I have to look forward to with regard to treatment, I am nevertheless calm about the whole situation. Bonnie seems to be doing well too.

See you here soon.

Chapter 5 - Maintaining What's Important

"Love is life. And if you miss love, you miss life."
~ Leo Buscaglia.

Monday, November 22, 2010 – Lesson from Life

Have you ever thought about what is important? I mean really important. Not your job, your office, not your car, your house, or any of your prestige or your things.

I mean what really matters. Most things you can lose, but replace. Some things you just can't replace, like someone you love.

People matter, and in particular, those people. The ones we love, the ones that love us, the people that depend on you, and the people you depend on. The people that love you, the people that give, support and share for nothing. They do so for no reason other than the kindness and love in their hearts. It is their desire to make your life better. To enrich all they touch. Because it is good, and it matters – to them, that you are comforted or happy, or pleased, or amused, or humored in some way.

Those people teach us to be better people. To hone our own contributions to be bigger and better, and more valuable as we learn to give without taking, because we learn to care and know that is the essence of what matters.

Where does this come from? Why do some people have it in large measure, and some people are just evil? Is it because of genetics? Maybe. Maybe not, it probably is a case-by-case reality. Some people are good and become great. Others are OK and become terrible.

I think a lot of the outcome ultimately, is up to each individual. You can't blame love or hate - on luck. People either strive to develop a relationship and to enrich it, ignore it because they are centered on something that doesn't really matter, or pour amazing amounts of energy into dark acts. Which is energy that could have just as easily been used for something good.

I expect when I get to the gates - God will know what my W2 looks like and won't care. God will know I had a Corvette and won't care. God will know my address and doesn't care. I believe the million dollar question also isn't what love did I get. I think the whole judgment is what love did you give with no expectation.

Did you stop to change the tire for that elderly couple? Did you make a difference more than not? Did you enrich the lives of your children, or give them an example of who they don't want to become? Did you enrich the life of your spouse, your siblings, your parents, your neighbors, your community, your colleagues, your place of worship? Are you learning from your mistakes in life? Are you honing who you are? Did you give enough? If not why not? Did the other things you were doing, really matter?

I know better now than ever, the importance of these things. I am facing mortality; does it take that to figure it out? Not for everyone. Others will never get it.

I believe the world is far more weighted toward good than evil. Unfortunately, the evil minority seems to have an unfair influence on the quality of life here on planet Earth. But whatever the driving reason is for evil people, I feel my life has been influenced more by the good spirit that you have, and have shared with me, and others.

I know that because you wouldn't have read this far if you weren't a loving, giving person.

It's people and all we love that matters.

My family, my dogs, my friends, my colleagues, the sunset, the Elk that drift though the 200 acre parcel across the street, Paul McCartney, Mozart, and a ton of other things that God influences to fill our hearts with joy. None of that costs anything, and yet it has the most value and in the end, is the only thing that really matters.

Before it is too late, did you make a difference today?

What did you give?

Did it really matter?

Monday, October 17, 2011 – Why Me Lord? I'm too young to go!

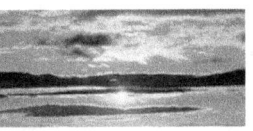

Confession time – I don't feel persecuted, picked on, or singled out. I do have cancer, and my doctor seems to think that it will kill me by and by. I can accept that. It seems ridiculous to believe that just because I have cancer that the rules don't apply to me. I am nobody special; there isn't any reason why cancer can't kill me.

But it brings up some interesting questions. It is because of my mortality that I have begun to think about all of this. It seems the more I think about it, the more perplexed I ultimately become.

Here's what I mean.

I believe in God. I believe that God can at least partially be explained as the energy that is the essence of everything and is collectively the consciousness of the almighty. To me this explains how God can be everywhere, know everything, hear our thoughts, turn water into wine, etc. So God is all, knows all, and can do anything. Do you believe that? I think it is more or less right.

So, is it God's fault that I have cancer? Did God make a decision to make it grow, or conversely make a decision to prevent it? Maybe. But I doubt either. Yet the conundrum gets even more complex for me. Here's why.

I think we could agree that God didn't give me cancer per se. Maybe it's like free will or like a river flowing. Some things just take their own path. Following the path of least resistance. I don't think God has anything to do with whether a river turns left or right. Nor do I think God is involved with whether I got or would not have gotten cancer. It simply is what it is.

We all know that God has unconditional love for all of us. So, if you had unlimited capabilities, would you standby and watch your child suffer a slow and not so pretty death to a disease like cancer? Or anything else for that matter? Have you ever wondered about this stuff? Why does God allow suffering for the children he loves unconditionally? I don't have the answer to that, do you?

But here is where my head takes this. First of all, I don't believe there is a clock in heaven. I believe that God knows all about inter-dimensional space where time doesn't exist. Our scientists are only just beginning to understand the fabric of space-time. But of course, God knows all about it nevertheless. God talks about those that arrive in heaven experiencing those that arrive later as arriving in what appeared to be a twinkling of an eye. Einstein talks about time and space as relative to the observer. But without going too deep into that, the point I am trying to make is that anyone suffering though a death here on Earth, may appear to an observer in heaven as a very short event. Maybe.

Another aspect to my confusion is by reference. For instance, look at all of the biblical characters that had a long or even extended amount of suffering they endured. God was OK with that; God was OK to watch his only son die a horrible death. One can conclude it doesn't matter. Not that he doesn't care. He has to care. It's just in the larger view, with eternity as a backdrop, it doesn't matter. If it did, people wouldn't die, nor would the critters around us.

On the other hand - a protracted and unpleasant death matters to me. Suffering through these things ultimately makes a difference to me. But, if you had the perspective from heaven, and time was always the same and never ending, would suffering though a death have the same significance?

Is it possible that the judgment of the character you have, while doing something difficult exposes what is really important to God and those in heaven? Is that the point?

Or is the point simply that it exposes you to very difficult circumstances which draws you closer to God. Maybe it is simply a wakeup call to prepare! How lucky is that? I have time to prepare everything before I die, including family, my friends, colleagues, and myself. It is much better than an instant and unexpected death.

At a different level, is the point of life just about learning lessons of right and wrong so that when you arrive in heaven you have a basis of personal understanding and appreciation for all that is good so you fit in? Probably.

Look, I don't think I have the answers. But I do think I am beginning to find a framework where some of this is making sense to me more than it ever has before.

Who knows what will happen. Maybe I have a miraculous healing, or maybe I die before I want to. I don't know. I firmly believe God has my best interests in mind. So I can relax and let the plan unfold.

This is not a capitulation muse. However, I am entering into a difficult second round of cancer. I am not as strong as I was the first time, or as confident. But I am nevertheless still strong in my commitment to do everything I can to get through this. I will take the medicine and work to heal.

Yet, the statistics aren't good. But who knows, maybe I will be the oddball that makes it through. If not, my life has been rich, I have loved and been loved and I have more friends that care about me than I deserve.

Someday we will all be in heaven, the mystery will be over, and we will know what a perfect existence is.

I'm looking forward to that.

Saturday, October 22, 2011 - Second Verse, Same as the First!

I can't say that I am looking forward or ready for this, but Wednesday is chemo day again.

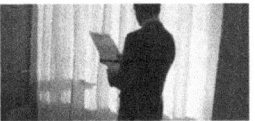

The first of many to come.

This stuff is nasty and it makes me feel like I have a bad flu. With chemo, I will start having flu like symptoms near the end of October, and that will stretch into February. That folks is definitely a drag.

Which of course is the down side.

On the bright side, I will get through it, although I will get banged up along the way - of course. Who knows - you can't be sure, but I am entering this round not as strong, so it may well be worse. But I will get through and I fully expect to drive this into remission a second time. I did it before, no reason to believe that I can't do it again.

The question of course is - will it stay gone, or will it come back to haunt me another time? I am hoping round two will be the knockout round. Keep your fingers crossed.

Another positive that may not be so obvious, it will make me feel better. My immunization system is really revved up right now trying to fight this cancer. So I don't have a lot of energy. And I just don't feel real well. If I allow myself to get tired, then I really pay for it, and it can take days to get better.

I guess nobody ever expects to go though this. It just happens. For sure it has had strong and powerful influence on me in a most positive way. I even think I needed it to get the wake up call in a number of different areas of personal development. Maybe there are larger even more valuable lessons waiting ahead. I don't know. Personally, I would like to just win and get on with what I perceive to be the valuable gifts of life.

Through this experience, I wish I could give everyone a picture of how lucky we are and how many blessing there are to be thankful for, in ways that could touch every heart.

But it seems these things have to be achieved individually and through experience. However, if I could, that would be my gift to human kind. A simple awareness of just how good things are in ways that would bring joy for you, and make the things that are otherwise annoying seem as small as they actually are.

So here's to life, may it bring blessings and happiness to you.

Saturday, October 29, 2011 – Same old Song, Grateful Nevertheless

Gratitude may seem odd, but I am.

I woke up this morning with nausea, and yet, I was listening to Bonnie singing, and making a great breakfast. I got up, took a shower, she had fresh biscuits, egg sandwiches, bacon, orange juice, coffee and a slug of vitamins ready. Bonnie, Marci and I had a really nice breakfast. I shared bacon with the dogs.

Later, the dogs were barking at the door, so I got up to check that, my friend Adrian had been to Apple Corporate, and sent me a cool Apple shirt, which was in a FedEx pack inside the door. After checking that out, I sat down to start writing this blog, the doorbell rang, this time it was Randy from Schwan's, delivering good food and good cheer. He talked about the Blog and people he knows that are reading it. We talked about things that are important in life; it was about people and good deeds.

So I am predictably ill from the chemo, and unpredictably grateful for the constant reminders of how many good people and good things there are that surround all of us. I have heard from so many people via text, email, Facebook, and calls. All with good cheer, high hopes and high spirits.

It is just impossible to tell you how much spirit that imparts and the value it plays for me. But it is huge, and I am grateful to all of you.

Cancer is evil, but it continues to contribute nourishment to my character and to my soul.

I am feeling stuck knowing that I have a long road ahead, and not feeling I have a choice. But we don't always get those options. This is the hand that has been dealt, and this is the one I will play as gracefully as I can. I refuse to sink into darkness, when there is so much light around, no matter what.

So I am sending hugs for all, to express my thanks and gratitude to friends that are forever and true.

Saturday, November 5, 2011 - Having Déjà vu, Wishing for Amnesia

The good news is that I am doing great! The bad news is I expect that to change. Chemo is cumulative, the longer you take it the more difficult it becomes.

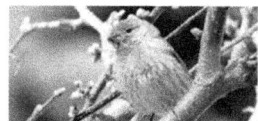
From my front yard

So I just got through round 1 of 8, had some issues, but feeling pretty good all in all. Hey its still poison, so it isn't easy, but really, I'm feeling pretty good.

Got a call from a personal friend who is a physician in Canada. We have been friends for some twenty years. You know, you just never know when or where the pearls are going to come from. Dr. Paul Farrel was asking me how I feel, so I told him the very abbreviated version. He actually already knows the details. I took it as more of a polite question.

Aren't friends priceless? He tells me, with all seriousness, that if I ever need to talk, day or night, three o'clock in the morning, whatever - whenever, to call. Now this is a guy that has more alphabet soup behind his name than anyone I have ever known. He is a practicing physician. People's aches and pains are his living. But somehow friendship transcends all of that, Paul is standing by for me because he is my friend not my doctor. God Bless you Paul, I'm sure God favors hearts as good as yours.

That was the pearl, but what about the wisdom? We started talking about the will to live, and the difference that makes. I mentioned that all of the medical types I have talked to have said that the key most important determining factor in the health of a cancer patient, is a strong positive attitude. In Paul's typical style with a brain that operates about 12 times faster than mine, he said, "the key most important factor is the raw determination to live."

Subtle difference, but powerfully different. One is an attitude, the other addresses ones will to survive.

Paul talked about a lady with Lymphoma who was told she had three months to live. 9 years later she is doing well, and still has Lymphoma. She simply refuses to capitulate. Isn't that awesome?

He talked about another guy that could have lived with a minor injury, who "unplugged" somehow and was dead in 8 hours.

Yet - God has the wheel. When he decides your time is up, your time is up.

For the rest of us, there are choices. It may boil down to one thing, how much do you want to live?

Is there anything so important to you that you can't let go of life?

If you believe in God and heaven, you know that it is eternal. For me, and for now, heaven can wait. I have a life to live, and commitments to fulfill. For certain, I have a rough road ahead, but not rougher than my resolve. I choose the life I am living.

Oh you will read about my complaints in this blog. I will have those inevitably. Yet, I believe in the hereafter, and think that is highly desirable.

But for now I also have a lot to live for – regardless of cancer or anything else.

I don't want to get to heaven by being a slacker!

I have work to do here and now - and there are people that count on me for a variety of things.

Thursday, November 10, 2011 - I Intend to Live Forever, So Far, so Good.

I have finished the second round of Chemo. On the plus side, the first round was not overly difficult, on the down side; the effects didn't completely go

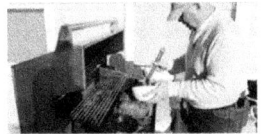

Prime Rib at Christmas

away. It is a fourteen-day cycle. To fight metastatic cancer, I get infused on every other Wednesday for about five to six hours. They give me a host of things, including three varieties of chemo:

1. *Fluorouracil (5-FU) (which interrupts the action of an enzyme that blocks synthesis of pyrimidine thymidine, which is a nucleotide required for DNA replication. That stunts growth. I also get leucovorin at the same time, a vitamin 'A' enhancement from folic acid which enhances the 5FU;*

2. *Camptosar (which keeps DNA from unwinding and therefore can't multiple) which prevents growth, it is a genetically targeted drug and;*

3. *Avastin, which is a drug that blocks angiogenesis, the growth of new blood vessels essentially used to prevent the supply of blood required for growing cancer.*

In cancer speak this treatment is known as "Full Fury."

In addition to the chemo, I also get a steroid to keep me somewhat healthy and functional. It is designed to pick me up from the impact of the poison. It lasts 48 hours. They give me Atropine to prevent cramping, and of course, an anti-nausea medication for me, as well as the medical staff that have to treat me; and my obnoxious attempts at humor and love.

I have four types of nausea meds at home, which work to cover each of the four-neuro pathways that can trigger nausea. All of this basically makes me feel kind of like having the flu. Big headaches, fatigue, poor appetite. Not to mention GI related issues.

When I leave the infusion center, they provide me with a battery-powered pump that connects to the port in my chest, which I carry around in a little black bag. That continues to infuse 5FU into me until Friday at noon, at which time I go to the hospital to have the pump taken off. Coincidently, that is also the time that the steroids wear off, and I crash into increasing levels of illness. They give me a liter of saline at that time to help flush poison out.

After I leave, I am basically worthless, do some work but then I am down through Saturday and in bed. Sunday I start moving around, and Monday I get up and work.

That may sound difficult, but it is manageable. Also, I consider work a blessing. It keeps me engaged in doing things that are good for my soul and me. Fortunately the people I work for like me, my contribution, and are happy with my work ethic, output at a Vice President level, and are fine with me doing it from home.

The problem with the round of chemo I just finished is that by the next weekend, when I would have expected to be basically up and at 'em, I was not.

I missed a close friends daughter's birthday party Friday night, and lunch out with my sister on Sunday. It is likely a combination of just getting physically worn down over a long period of time, having my immunization system revved up and fighting cancer which is tiring, and getting large doses of what is effectively poison all of which just makes me ill folks.

After careful consideration I have come to the well-considered conclusion that cancer sucks. Not only for those that have it, but for all that are impacted by it as well. OK – so that was definitely what my friends in the UK and it's colonies (you know who you are), would call whinging (whinge - an informal verb. To complain, moan, grumble, grouse, gripe). I think I am allowed some of that. It is some more of the brutal truth).

However, I would never close on that note.

Spiritually I am fine. I have said it before and I will say it again, my body is ill, everything in my brain is doing just fine. I am happy, hopeful, positive, humored, contributing, loved and loving, excited, and most of all grateful to God, and in the same breathe grateful to all of the family and friends that support me.

I have said this before also, and I will say it again as well. You make a difference. All of you plus my family lift me up and give me the will to carry on.

If you read my last blog, you also know just how strong my will to live - continues to be.

I feel compelled to say that my will to live is because I feel obligated more to life and all it brings, than to taking the easy way out, and having a great high-end vacation that goes on in perpetuity with some really nice people in a really great place.

Here's my Salute to life, and honor for God who provides it.

Thanks to all of you, that have taken the role of self-appointed guardian soldiers. You rock.

It will come back to you. It always does.

Saturday, November 19, 2011 - Believe you can and . . . You're halfway there

I had a good week, I hope you did too!

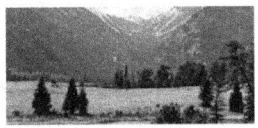

Rocky Mountain
National Park

From a cancer point of view, my big issue all week was nausea. Gee, I wonder why? When I saw my oncologist Sam last week, he had just finished filling a large vessel in the back of his building with rat poison. My advice, do yourself a favor and skip the whole cancer experience. Unless you just think you need to have a major character building exercise. One thing is for sure; it will either build your character or destroy it and kill you at the same time!

Even though I would have selected option A, - no cancer (if I had been given the option), I also know that it has been one of the better gifts I have ever received. That sounds strange to hear, even as I am thinking it. Yet sometimes reality is stranger than fiction.

If I do a little self-analysis and pardon me for saying it, but I have always been a bit of a brainiac - I am not referring to any degree of intelligence, I am saying that when I have self evaluated myself in the past, I have always been very grateful for my interest in everything, ability to learn, as well as remember things. All of that followed by an ability to deductively use new knowledge. In my value system, that has always been something I have been very grateful for. It is the reason I have the life that I do with all it brings. What a treasure.

However, learning things and being able to use that knowledge, doesn't have a lot to do with social skills. For many years I focused on the collection of knowledge. Again, I am not unhappy about that, I am in fact grateful for all that it provided. Yet in full health, and in full living stride, the opportunity never really arose to think about more of the human and spiritual issues that are so important.

In reading this book, you already know that I have had a transformation in values. The last year has lead to prioritization around the human experience. That doesn't mean I have abandoned the intellectual pursuit. As an example, last week I spent three days working a very complex spreadsheet to calculate any video format, with multiple variables through time, to understand how much storage capacity is required. It is very mental work and I love that stuff. Yet, at the end of the day my thoughts and prayers are about humanity.

I believe that gives me an important balance as a human. I doubt I would have ever achieved the acuity of thought on humanity and spiritual awakening I have now, had it not been for the cancer I now battle. Because I now believe the priority of life is about human compassion, I therefore believe the cancer experience has been the vessel that has carried me to a new level of awakening. For that, I am grateful. I think this is work in progress by they way, and that gives me a sense of joy, for knowing the best is yet to come.

It all starts as a life experience that leads to a thought that paves the way to a human awakening.

God provides these opportunities in many ways, most of them are fairly stressful it seems.

If what you are getting out of these stressful opportunities is anguish, I would suggest you might be missing the opportunity.

Walt Disney once said, "If you can dream it, it can come true."

Theodore Roosevelt said, "Believe you can and your halfway there."

I believe I am in round two for the battle of my life, and I am halfway there. Where does that take me? To a place that has opened my heart, and my spirit. The greatest gift one can receive, which I will treasure for the rest of my life.

It is only because of this experience, that I will be honing myself for what happens next.

What do you believe in?

Friday, November 25, 2011 - It sucks to be me

OK don't get excited, just some wicked perspective coming your way.

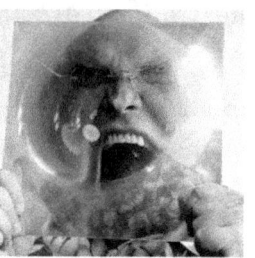

"Randy"
Photo by
Jamie Hurt

So let's see. 0400 Sunday morning I woke up shriving as if I had a serious dunk in a cold lake and was hypothermic. I turned the electric blanket on 1. When my teeth started rattling, I decided I needed more heat, so I bumped it to 3. No good, I just got worse. I reached out and touched Bonnie - she asked what was wrong? I told her I was freezing; she bumped the heat to 9!

We waited but alas, no joy. I'm telling you I was <u>COLD</u>. She took my temp. Normal. She took my blood pressure, 182/104. Mhhhhh? Time to call 911. 15 minutes later we have an ambulance, and fire truck in the driveway.

Next thing you know, I have eight people in my bedroom. One of the paramedics approached the side of the bed, Roxy, lying next to me, snarled and lunged at the guy. Oops! "It's OK Roxy, lay down," which she did. Abby was barking from her kennel. Bonnie told her "<u>NO</u>!" she instantly stopped. Pretty cool.

Then we start playing twenty questions. No, no, no, no, you get the drill. The paramedic that was in charge, says, "Well we can transport you to the hospital." I told her I didn't need another ride in an ambulance, or a visit to the hospital to feel complete, so with no fear that I was heading toward a cliff, they left.

Eventually I stopped shaking, but did a Rip Van Winkle act all day on Sunday. They told me to call my Doctor on Monday, but heck, why do that? Everything seemed OK by Monday. Besides, who wants to moan and groan. I have serious issues to think about, I didn't need to add trivial complaints. So I ignored it.

Monday was Monday, so I got up at 6am and went to work. I have to. I set up my MBOs to deliver three alliances by December 24th, three white papers, and three presentations to support each of the three alliances with a host of other things to do on top of that.

However, I couldn't get to that work because I had a nagging bug in a VERY complex spreadsheet used to calculate any video format, with about 5 other variables, to how much storage is required over what period of time for a selection of any of our products. That was a brainteaser and a half, but I finally got it worked out. With that done, I wanted to get back to writing the complex white paper, which I won't even begin to describe, but had to first review a paper written by another analyst.

Meanwhile, we get confirmation that the inspections and the appraisal went through on the sale of our house, so we are moving to closing. Yeah, no problem. Now I'm thinking about the mountain of stuff I have to move while being ill from chemo, and carry my load at work.

I decided I am going to skip chemo the week of December 16th, because that is when we start this parade from where we live to the new house. In a neighborhood. With neighbors, something we haven't done in about 24 years. Someone needs to warn "the neighbors" about me.

Of course you know this is Thanksgiving week, and I above many, have lots to be thankful for. As it turns out, Thanksgiving is also our son David's birthday. He drove up from near Santa Fe, and arrived about three in the afternoon Wednesday.

I had a really productive day on the white paper I was writing. Dogs start barking, and David comes in. About the same time a wave of nausea sweeps over me. 10 minutes later, I'm shivering again. Gee, maybe I should have called Sam, my oncologist, on Monday, naa – I'm not a baby. Nevertheless, I thought I would call Sam, just to prevent Bonnie from calling out the 911 dogs again. Sam's staff invited me to come in and have a nice little visit – stat.

OK great, let's go see Sam. Bottom line, they drew blood and Sam seriously dressed me down. It's what you don't know that will kill you when you have cancer. The concern was that the chemo had shut off my immunization system. A blood draw and what they call a Complete Blood Count (CBC) would show what the white blood cell count is, and whether it had cratered. The shivering is because I have some sort of infection, a very dangerous problem when your immunization system is shut down, Sam was pleasantly very unhappy with me, and made it

*clear, including unveiled threats of violence –
seriously.*

*Sam sends me home, and calls about two hours later
to let me know that I was OK, my white blood cell
count has not cratered, and the new antibiotics
should do the trick. In case I missed his dressing
down in the office, he did it again on the phone. I
simply said, "Yes sir." I love Sam.*

I have chemo coming up again next Wednesday.

*I have alliances, presentations, and white papers to
write, while I am managing certification and
benchmarks on new products to complete by
Christmas.*

We are moving the week of December 16th.

The pressure is on.

Now you know why it sucks to be me.

*Count you blessing for your health, and the health of
all that you love. It makes getting through life
easier. A lot easier.*

*And oh by the way, I don't care. I'm getting though
this, just to prove how stubborn I really am.
Cancer? No problem, bring it on. I'm beginning to
like chemo.*

"Another chemo please." – Thank you.

I'm lucky to be alive.

Chapter 6 - Inner Strength

"The weaker I become physically, the stronger I become inside."

Saturday, December 3, 2011 - You miss 100% . . . of the shots you don't take
Wayne Gretzky said it, and I agree.

I have taken some shots that have resulted in getting hit in the head by Thor's hammer it seems. But I don't think I have left a lot on the ice. I have won and I have lost – big, in each direction.

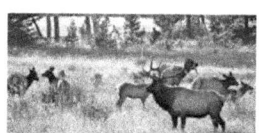

Elk in Rocky Mountain National Park

But even the losses have at some point felt like victories. Because from each of them I have refined a lack of something, character, compassion, understandings, patience, empathy, knowledge, etc. It's all good sooner or later.

People keep asking me how I am. It seems that just because I have a terminal (at some point) disease, that I must be emotionally bush-wacked. Seriously folks, I'm not.

Even if I was on my deathbed, I'm not going to be racked with regrets or sadness that matter. You will never hear me saying, "I could have done this, and I should have done that."

Regardless of how right or wrong I have been, to me, the path has always been good. I hope your choices have been good for you too. I have played the game of life with heart and I am happy with the results.

Have you ever noticed that what appears at first to be a big issue, after things play out – eventually turns into a good experience if not a really positive one? It has always been that way for me, countless times. Perception has a lot to do with it, and realizing that the opportunities that exist today, would not have happened in any other way. I hope you see and appreciate this as well.

This is chemo week. I expect to be sick. At the same time, I expect to be better, because I am just unwilling to be robbed of life. Not today or tomorrow. The reality is that the robustness of my life has diminished with cancer. The disease has limited my options. I have missed some important events, and I will miss more of them.

But I am in the fast lane with the cards I have been dealt. Example, if you have know me then you also know that I have been an amateur photographer since I was a teenager. This week I did a major upgrade. I bought a much better digital SLR Nikon camera. I expect to be able to accomplish better photographs with a better tool. I am planning success in photography.

I am planning success in work, I am planning success at home, and I expect to win this round of cancer.

My kind advice, if you or someone near you has cancer, don't let the people who don't have it influence you into believing that you are finished.

I firmly believe that your faith, spirit, and commitment will carry you beyond the statistical boundaries you get from the doctors, and expectations that others may have.

It's game time folks - take the shot. Choose to live, and to refine who you are and what your contribution is along the way from the rich experiences that life offers.

If you don't have cancer, still - take the shot. You won't always be in the position to do so. You can set yourself on a path that leads to a position that allows you to "take the shot". Creating the opportunity to make a difference to the people you love is priority number one.

The shot you take should benefit all of them, and you.

Saturday, December 10, 2011 - There's no next time, It's now or never.

I am reminded once again how. I had a great night out last night trying out my new Nikon, with some dear friends that were attending a high school wrestling match their son was participating in.

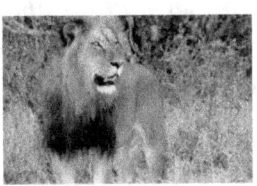

In South Africa

Young people everywhere, and energy was high for everyone. I had a great time shooting pictures of Cameron McCrimmon, a terrific person and talented young athlete. I was lucky to be sitting with Clifton and Heather his Father and Mother, and brother Austin. All people I think the world of.

About eight o'clock I went home, and watched Cowboys and Aliens with the family. It was a really fun movie.

When I got up from that, my kidneys started hurting really bad. So it was off to the hospital at about 10:30 pm. I was in ER until about 0600 Saturday morning, when they admitted me. I am here now writing this.

The good news is that they haven't found anything really wrong, and they know the cancer in my lungs is diminishing based on the CT scan they did last night. The bad news is they can't really explain the pain. I will be here at least through tonight.

The staff here is tripping over themselves to help me, and make me feel better.

Last week I got a call from a dear friend to let me know that I am in her mind, and that I am loved. Camberley Bates has been a champion friend to me. Another call from Kris Phillips, same thing – she was checking in and making sure I am OK. Our families are going to celebrate when I go into remission. Gary Francis called because he cares.

We are moving next week. Ron McCrimmon sent email and wants to know what time to be there. Not, can I help, no – what time do I need to be there? Brian Bates is coming over to help me organize my garage along with Ron. A colleague, Jeff's little boy, is praying for me at bedtime.

Again, how many great people are there in the world? The supply seems to be endless. The world is full of people that care from their very soul and heart. It's easy to be depressed with the daily newscasts and be overwhelmed by the evil doings of the more sinister side of humanity. There seems to be an ample supply of that as well.

But let me tell you humanity at large is good, and this cancer is a blessing. Most people will never know the amount of people that care for them, in measures that are no less than startling.

Something I did for someone, simply because I could, that made a difference to them. A real difference. I may not remember, but they do. Boy do people remember, and they want me to know. I have been to funerals where all of that is being poured out in eulogy. The person being honored and remembered may have never had a chance to hear it, or feel it, or experience the unbridled love of humanity. But I have, and I didn't have to die to find out. To me, that makes cancer a blessing.

Life is real - this isn't a practice session. There is no next time, it's now or never. You may be the recipient of good deeds, you may be the giver, either way it is good, and you should engage to do good things often, because it makes a difference.

Once again, I thank all of you for making a difference to me. I am humbled and honored beyond measure.

Thursday, December 29, 2011 - "Courage to stand up and speak - Courage to sit down and listen."

The full quote is: "Courage is what it takes to stand up and speak; courage is also what it takes to sit down and listen."   *- Winston Churchill*

Remember when the lion from the Wizard of Oz was looking for courage? In the end you find out that he had it all along.

Courage is in you.

General Randy

"Success is not final, failure is not fatal: it is the courage to continue that counts."

- Winston Churchill

I believe I have to continue. On the other hand, I don't feel courageous. I feel obligated, hopeful, and most of all grateful for so many things.

However, other people have commented on my courage. But what is courage? Am I courageous simply because I have not given up or in? Some people would accuse me of just being stubborn. I don't feel that is exactly it. I just feel dedicated to live up to my responsibilities to God, Family, friends and colleagues.

Hanging around with the cancer community, I have found there are some that believe way too much in the Doctors. Don't get me wrong, I love and admire the medical teams I have been subjected to. But you have to listen to <u>everything</u> they say. Sure they will give you probabilities for success and failure. But *those statistics are not death sentences. At least they are not intended to be.*

Yet, I hear story after story of people that throw in the towel upon receiving dour news. Why? Is it because they believe the doctors so much that they instantly know they will soon die? Which is really odd because the doctors are not sending that message. Or is it because they are so unhappy with other elements in their lives they can use the big "C" as the reason to checkout?

I don't know, I don't have all the answers. There are too many people and individual circumstances to know for sure. But I do know this. I have known of people that have died within hours of receiving the news that they have a tough cancer. I also know of people that have lived more that 10 years after receiving news they would statistically die within a year.

The difference is in the individual.

More than anything else you have to trust the medical team to do the right things, you have to believe in yourself, and maintain a strong will to live for what drives you.

I don't know how you feel about intuition. I can tell you that in my life I have had some amazing intuitive insights. You know that voice that speaks to you? Well yesterday, the day before I went in for chemo, I had the voice tell me I was going to be fine. And that is what I believe. I will be fine.

It's been a rough road folks. I was more ill yesterday on this most recent round than ever before. I am feeling a significantly better today and will gradually climb out of this hole.

It has been a strenuous two weeks since I last posted a blog. We have moved and are in out new home. We have been unpacking like crazy. We had Christmas and a full house to entertain and look after. This week was a chemo week. All of which is enough to take a toll on me. On top of that Bonnie was ill. However and on the bright side, we all had fun, I have enjoyed my family, and heard from many dear friends around the world. I am very grateful for that.

I have a PET Scan coming up in a couple of weeks to find out how mean mister cancer is doing, so I will let you know about that. I already know that it is diminishing from the CT scan a couple of weeks ago, so I expect good news.

By the way, I get a lot of courage from all of you. Courage to stand up and speak. I get a lot of Courage from Sam (my oncologist) where I sit down and listen. Bonnie and I think together, I believe in Sam, God, Bonnie's good care and your love. I am fine now, and I am going to get better.

Love to all of you.

Time to Retire

It was just getting to hard to keep up with the workload and have enough time to rest and heal. As a result, I moved from employment to retirement. That was made easier by short-term, and then long-term disability insurance, as well as government disability, which I am now on.

Saturday, January 7, 2012 - Things that were hard to bear, are sweet to remember

Everything I seem to fret over turns into a blessing. I wish I knew that ahead of each worry. As luck would have it, I am finally beginning to think about it ahead of time, which leaves me a much happier person.

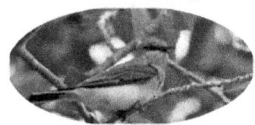

In my back yard

Today is a day that is filled with thinking of the past. Especially the wonderful fortune I have had during my career. Prompting this reflection comes from taking the final step to retire yesterday, 1/6/12. Yes, I have hung up my spurs. It comes with a degree of confusion and regret, yet I am excited and hopeful.

There are so many facets of the joy I have experienced throughout the career journey. Most of it has been about great friendships that continue to span great distances and have endured many years. In a number of cases the friendships have more significance than just a pal. People that I feel connected to. People that I have laughed and cried with. People I call brothers and sisters because their significance, hits me at an emotional level equal to my family.

Through good fortune I have relationships with people that stretch though 40 years of a working career and includes every continent.

Another aspect of fulfillment has been the work. I have not gone to work daily for that many years unhappily. I have loved the mental challenge of understanding complex ideas, and translating them into cogent perspective and value. For some I suppose that would be horrible, for me it has just been a delight, full of rewarding joy.

Of course there have been difficult challenges, but from them I have grown, learned, and adapted. Ultimately strengthening what I have to offer and the person I am. It seems the mistakes and failures along the way all lead to a success. The failures seem to be hard lessons in disguise, leading to growth that results in some value.

So, with a degree of regret and concern for not having anymore starring moments, I have chosen to put healing and family first. Bonnie desires more time with me, more than she cares about the possibility that I accomplish another notch in my career gun. Likewise, she is more important to me than the next work related breakthrough. So for all of you that I know and have worked with, I love you all. Thanks for making my life richer.

For the first time in forty years, I wake up Monday with no action items from work. The major thing I have to accomplish on Monday is completing some disability paperwork, and a PET scan to check on the progress of cancer. I already know it will be good news. The cancer is in retreat; it is only a question of how good the news will be.

I had one more episode of bilateral kidney pain this week. This time I just called the doc to make sure I am not being stoically stupid, rationalized it on the phone, I didn't go in, and basically just toughed it out for a day and a half. Here's a heads up for you. You don't get any rest in a hospital. There are too many busy bodies taking care of you.

Final thoughts for the week:

I am so lucky. I can't even begin to enumerate it. Angels surround Bonnie and I, God seems to sit on my shoulders, everything that causes me angst, is a step toward God making my life better. I'm giving up. I may as well turn the keys over and just believe that everything I want to worry over is handled. That said, all I have to worry about is getting over cancer, and even that, I ultimately believe will also be OK.

If there is one business opportunity I have missed, it is in finding a way to bottle my luck and good fortune. I am just humbled and grateful for it, and all of you.

By the way, you may wonder what I am going to do to keep my brain engaged.

One thing I would like to do is to attend a culinary academy.

Something I am going to do is write a book:

"Prospering with Cancer – Finding the Joyful and Valued Lessons Cancer Provides.

Maybe I can help others though the difficult parts of their journey.

God Bless all of you.

Tuesday, January 10, 2012 - There is no education Like Adversity

On Monday I got the PET scan, and of course, brought the radiology home to "read" it. We all know I am unqualified, but why should I let that get in my way?

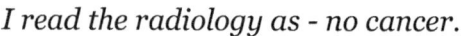

I read the radiology as - no cancer.

Just saw Sam today. Fortunately - he agrees. I have no metabolically active cancer.

I don't know what the plan is yet, I will find out tomorrow.

More to come . . .

I am so amazed at where all of this has led me, and what I have learned.

God is still taking care of us.

Saturday, January 14, 2012 - Live your beliefs and you can turn the world around

"Live your beliefs and you can turn the world around".
~ Henry David Thoreau

I believe in the power of prayer, love, support, and even my own will. All of these things have carried me through one of life's more difficult challenges, terminal cancer. Any event that is life threatening is challenging. It impacts the person with the challenge of living, 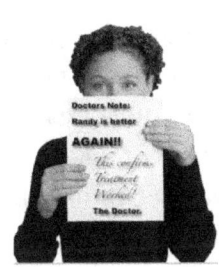 *but also a large surrounding circle of people that care. Each of them look for solace and healing, at the same time they offer love, support, and prayers.*

Your love and support has come in many different ways. I believe that all of these things contributed to my healing.

In order of priority I believe God's will is number one. Ultimately I feel like a passenger on God's bus. I don't know what curves or bumps are ahead, I just have to trust that God is driving me in the right direction. I also believe it is up to me to pay attention to try to understand where we are going, and try to play a supporting role in whatever God's will may be.

In the very beginning of this I felt that God provided cancer as a way to pull me into faith, and he wanted me to use my communication skills to help others in ways that I may be able to. At that time, I felt that was going to manifest itself by way of standup speaking engagements talking about finding the positive lesson that come with great challenges.

Now I believe that it is about writing a book. As a result, I will take the blogs that I have been writing for the last year and a half and use them as the guide posts for what needs to be written. If this is divine intervention, then I expect I will also get guidance on how the book should be written, the priority of message etc. So, if it is a success and winds up being helpful, glory to God. If it falls on it's face – shame on me. Either way, I will start soon.

The second priority is living your beliefs. I have managed to stay positive, find positive lessons, and carry out my life nearly normally from an outward appearance point of view. I have said many times, my body is ill, I am fine. However and inevitably, I have had doubtful and dark thinking moments. But each time that has come up, with prayer I have been able to quickly shake it off and move on with the more positive lessons and rewards of life through the experience. Surprisingly, some of the darkest moments have brought the brightest insights, lessons, and faith enriching moments.

My faith in God has expanded richly as has my commitment to healing. Pure faith and belief. It has helped me over the rough parts of being more ill than I have ever been in my life, and as ill as most people will ever get. I wish nobody the same experience, but I also know now that great challenges bring great and valuable insights, as well as emotional and spiritual rewards. I am lucky to have won two rounds of cancer.

I have no doubt that it will eventually kill me. But I will have benefited from the insights offered from humanity and God, which I would have never otherwise have received. I also hope that I can write a book that is helpful to others. I don't think I can overstate how valuable both God and humanity is to me.

Therefore, if I can use that experience to help others through what can potentially be a dark journey, than I think that purpose of my life will have been fulfilled along with being as good of a husband, father, friend and colleague as I can.

I believe life-threatening challenges makes it much easier to fall into the depths of despair. Without a foundation for belief and conviction, what else is there? Whether a person enters a difficult challenge with faith and belief, or finds it along the way, one must find it.

The power of healing lies there. The healing outcome is directly linked to faith and belief. Of course good medical care makes a difference. But, as I have mentioned before, two people with similar situations, one dies in hours, the other simply refuses to die. Faith and belief make a difference.

The prayers and support that all of you have given me has strengthened my resolve along the way and has been invaluable. It has given me a sense of responsibility to not let anyone down, and to feel worthy of what was freely given. That may sound odd, but it is true. Likewise, I continue to carry a sense of responsibility to God, to offer perspective that may help others to see their way through the challenge, avoiding despair, and to get through it as comfortably as possible, for them.

I believe dying is the greatest moment of life. I see it as graduation day. If you have lived the right life, believed and acted according to your faith, you are destined for heaven, and what could be better than that? At that time, the question is, are you living unfinished business? If death is known to be in your visible future, it certainly offers you time to get everything that needs to be taken care of finished. That is a blessing.

Perhaps one should feel an even a greater sense of responsibilities for affairs if you have no vision of dying, because it could happen fast, and it is permanent here on Earth.

Whatever your situation is, faith in God and belief in yourself are important.

God, all of you, my family, the medical team, and my faith have saved my life for now. I owe humanity a book and I am indebted to you, the people that made a tangible difference to my own resolve, faith and belief.

How can "thank you" cover that? Nevertheless – a heartfelt thanks.

For now, I am going to live a bit longer and try to make a difference.

Wednesday, January 25, 2012 - Every man dies. Not every man really lives

"Every man dies. Not every man really lives".

– William Ross Wallace

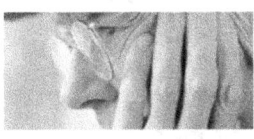

Today I am taking a major step toward living on. Today is the final installment of Chemo for this cycle.

I have beaten the cancer beast back twice now. I am in complete remission now. The last chemo treatment, and this one are all about mopping up any residual cancer that may be wandering around my body looking for mischief.

I feel inwardly quiet about this, not a jumping - arms up, shout of exuberance in celebration of winning round two. It is more a reflective feeling of what I have been through mentally, emotionally, spiritually, and physically.

I am sure we all have a different path to go down. For me, this has been the largest growth path of my life. It has awakened so much in me related not only to myself but also in understanding more of humanity and spirituality. I am sure there is far more to know than I already do, but I have nevertheless gained a lot.

With all of these virtues and values on the front of my mind, I sit and prepare myself to go in and take another shot in the final round of this battle. I am keenly aware as good as I feel now, by the time I come home around 3pm I will be quite ill again.

Mentally it is an exercise to steel up and get through. But I am alive, and I am grateful for it. I have enjoyed a rich experience here on our cozy planet, and I have living, learning, and loving yet to live. I have lived well, and I will continue for some time going forward.

I hope to return some of the rewards that have been given to me.

Round Three

I had a six-month respite from treatment. Although around the 4-month time frame I knew it was returning. Among my symptoms were an increase in fatigue and nausea, which were returning.

Bonnie and I have from nearly the beginning of our lives together dreamed of taking an RV trip across America in our retirement. Even though I knew cancer was returning, in May of this year we took a trip to explore Montana's rich environment. I could only drive about four hours a day, and we had to rest for a few days at a time so I could recover. But we made it through and had an awesome time.

When we returned, I had to go in for another PET scan, and got confirmation that I was facing the third round of cancer. It was active again in both my lungs and in my rectum.

Thursday, June 7, 2012 - Uncertainty is the only certainty

It has been a nice respite from Cancer over the last six months, but the ugly march has started again.

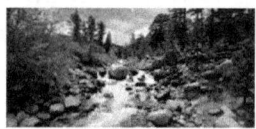

In Rocky Mountain National Park

I had a PET scan yesterday, and got the results today, it's back in both my rectum and in my lungs.

The plan is simple, the mix of chemo I have been having success with is recommended, and so I will begin that next week for a scheduled six cycles.

I pretty much knew it was back based on the way I was feeling. I will get through this one too, but truly friends, eventually this will kill me – the timing is of course uncertain. I could make it through years of this, or it could spread somewhere more critical, and I could be gone in a relatively short period of time. Time will tell.

In the meanwhile, chemo begins and with it will come the ups and downs of working to tolerate large doses of poison.

I will begin to write again to keep you posted on the journey.

Thank God for the health of all you love, and pray that it stays that way for as long as possible.

Wednesday, June 13, 2012 - Making stepping stones out of stumbling blocks

We all know that cancer is a struggle, it is filled with uncertainty and doubts for all that are subjected to its seemingly relentless march. I

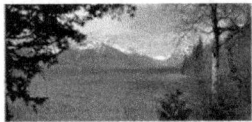

Glacier National Park

am entering the third stage of the battle for my life this morning. How would you feel?

I can tell you how I feel. Mostly normal. Sure I don't want to go in, take the poison and be sick – who would? But my state of mind is basically at rest and balanced. I believe, for the most part, it has been from the beginning.

The reason is that from the beginning I saw this as an issue that is much larger than I can deal with. So I prayed, telling God you have this one, I'm not going to worry about it, I will have to trust you to take care of it, and then I just let it go.

Amazingly enough, there have been moments, from time to time, that have been very stressful and worrisome. Yet, in each one of those challenging times, within days the solution appears and the situation resolves.

Today is another step toward a solution unknown to me. It's a bit like being on a passenger jet with an unknown destination – and not caring because you have enough faith to know the outcome will be all right, even though there are bumps along the way.

So – bon voyage, here I go again.

Saturday, June 16, 2012 - "If you're going through hell, keep going."

You may rest assured knowing that chemo hasn't changed. Its still poison, and it still makes one ill. Most of the time, consistency in experience is comforting for me, however – this is not.

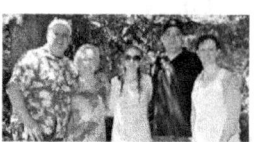

Randy, Bonnie, Marci, David, and Kim

On the other hand, I suspect that the chemo will do its evil work, and I will beat round three of this battle. I have been doing a little predictive analysis, if all factors remain constant; I believe I will be in remission once more after 4 rounds. That's the good news. The bad news is that I don't expect the battle to end.

It's just going to be a roller coaster ride. Beat it, and then it comes back – eventually, directly or indirectly, it kills me. By the way, I am not being down or negative here, that's what the experts tell me - and that's what I expect will happen.

Yea, yea, I know, miracles can happen, new drugs, etc. Just remember, the disease isn't waiting.

So, as Winston Churchill suggested, "while going through hell", I will just keep going. I think the best I can do is enjoy each day and contribute where I can.

I have finished my initial study of the Old Testament; I have to finish the New Testament now. If I am still going (and there is no reason to believe I won't at the moment), I will then start the book I want to write, "Prospering with Cancer".

Of course I will continue to enjoy photography too, which I will share.

The bottom line is this; I can deal with all the physical hassles of being ill and then not, and then again.

Yet, I can also carry on with enjoying some personal interests, and loving my family and friends at the same time. When you look at it that way, it looks pretty good eh? It does to me, because believe me, things could be worse, a lot worse.

The fact that I have a relatively easy path here - is a comfort.

And by the way - Thanks to Bonnie, who watches me like a hawk and nurtures me like a Saint.

Saturday, June 30, 2012 - God, Family, Friends, Cameras, and Computers.

"It is never too late to be what you might have been."

I've had a tough week. First it has been difficult to feel the mortality of my situation. I have already beaten the statistical odds of survival. Originally the doctors said a year to a year and a half. I am approaching two years since then. That has left me feeling like I am living on browed time going forward.

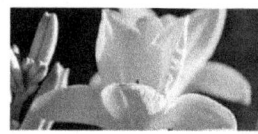
Tulip in my front yard

Bonnie and I just came back from a great month of RVing and sight seeing some of our nation's greatest splendors. The stuff we planned to do for a retirement for many years. While it was great, coming home to the news that I am active with cancer again was a downer. It is not a good sign to keep having it come back so rapidly. That decreases my chances of long-term survival. So that weighed heavy on me.

Last Saturday, I got up thinking about round two of chemo coming up on Wednesday of this week. Truthfully, I finally caught myself and realized I was just feeling sorry for myself. I don't want to let myself get into that mode of thinking.

So I asked myself, what's important? The answer came immediately, it is one we all already know, and I have a particular spin for - God, Family, Friends, Cameras, and Computers!

OK most everything is obvious. Let me explain my view. Certainly nothing is as important as God in your eternal life. God also directs that we love family, and our friends like family. I'm good with all of that.

However, when it comes to day-to-day joy of doing things, for me what's left is cameras and computers. I can capture the abundant beauty around us with my camera, and my computers allow me to manipulate them, but more than anything computers are a communications tool, which is grand.

You know, cancer is going to kill me. It could happen soon or I may have a few years. I just don't know. But I am refusing to succumb to dark thinking and self-absorbed pity. So I will get up when I am ill and I will work on my computer or take pictures or do something to enjoy the parts of life that I can, without worrying about long term horizons for what I may someday do.

I am relieved of any work related duties, so I really can just be in the moment with the things that are important to me. I have finished my initial study of the Old Testament and have a good start in the new. I still want to write a book called – "Prospering with Cancer", which I told myself I would do after I finish reading the Bible and having a reasonable working knowledge in it.

So while I feel I slipped off the shelf a bit in the beginning of the week, I think I am solidly back on it now.

I will also be working on rebuilding my web site so I can bring comments back.

God's blessing to each of you.

Sunday, July 8, 2012 - The Gift of Cancer

As this skirmish progresses, so do my thoughts. On the human side of the equation I often feel quite ill. Because of that I am unable to do many of the things I want to do. Like yesterday while in the

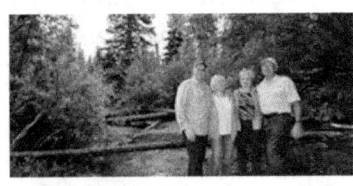

Randy, Bonnie, Sis, and Ray

mountains with family, I was unable to take a short walk they went on. I couldn't drive home, Bonnie had to. While she was driving my eyes were closed and I was leaning back in the chair just trying to maintain composure. I spent the rest of the day in bed initially waiting for the nausea meds to catch up, and then too fatigued to do anything.

If I allow myself, I could get angry, or depressed for what I have lost.

What I thought about was the beauty of a freshly rained forest, and how blessed I am to have the family I do. I got to take the camera out, and capture some great images of us together. That evening I learned that a dear friend who has suffered greatly by God's guiding hand was delivered yet another agonizing blow, along the path that is refining my friend to be one of the greatest servants to humanity I know.

These great challenges God delivers will either raise us or bury us. It is natural to ask the almighty why? But the question is not for what has been taken away, but for what growth and opportunity lies ahead.

Day to day I am suffering the physical effect of a progressive terminal disease; spiritually I am progressively refining my understanding of the lessons it teaches. I am far richer in my soul, than I was two years ago, I have found more happiness, love, and spirit than I have known at any other point in my life. God's greatest gifts are for the strong and faithful. No challenges are handed out that are designed to crush you, rather to strengthen, broaden, and heal you for the eternal person you must become.

Every day is precious to me, I thank God for the guidance and the great affinity for love I can share with family and friends. I pray your challenges lead you to better days always.

Saturday, July 14, 2012 - We can't control the wind, we can control our sails.

Cancer is a game of patience, faith, and hope. For some when cancer comes, emotional and physical battles are fought and 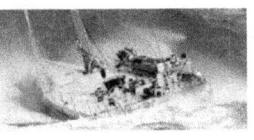 *won, it is then over, and people move on. Others have the experience of multiple bouts they eventually win, and still others have multiple bouts and lose their life.*

The patience game is trying to figure out where you are in the game, and not getting too messed up emotionally or physically while you wait, are taking lots of drugs, and feeling icky.

For me, having total confidence in our heavenly father has provided the patience and hope I need to feel balanced mentally, spiritually, and even physically. Without that I can't imagine where I would be. I turned this battle over very early on and it made a difference. It is quite amazing how so many things just worked out for the benefit of Bonnie and I.

It is difficult to not be hopeful that this new drug Sam is telling me about, is the silver bullet I need to survive. I think about how nice it would be to regain strength and health, get off disability, and go back to work.

In the meanwhile, Bonnie managed to find a deal to sell our truck and trailer, which were too large for her to handle, and trade them in for another diesel-pusher motor home, which she can handle.

She says she is going to go get it, bring it home, pack it, and tell me - let's go wherever for a few days. She is gutsy and bossy, but she keeps me going, laughing, and alive. We haven't even taken delivery of it yet, and she just booked a trip for Estes Park next week for a shakeout cruise.

With Bonnie all my friends, and Gods loving care, the wind randomly blows challenges my way, but my patience, faith, and hope remain solidly in play, for a course heading to success.

I wish God's blessing for all of you too.

Monday, July 23, 2012 - Beaten on the outside, stronger inside

Tomorrow I get another PET scan to determine my cancer status in round three of this battle with cancer. When cancer is active in me, one of the symptoms is

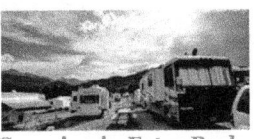

Camping in Estes Park

perpetual nausea. There are four pathways in a brain that can each trigger nausea. I have a medication for each, so I am able to manage it reasonably well. In the last two weeks, outside of the chemo treatment itself, I have had no nausea. My energy level has increased, and I have had a few days of feeling pretty good.

This gives me great hope that I will be, or nearly be in remission again. I will get the PET scan tomorrow, and of course, rush home to read the radiology myself. I will get the official results Wednesday, and will also likely get an amended plan for completion of this cycle of chemo. Even if cancer is gone, I expect to have to take another round for mop up reasons.

I am concerned about one thing. My lungs at times ache. I don't see that as good news, but again the PET scan will tell the story.

Overall, I have never been so physically beaten up in my life. I am very fatigued, with low endurance for much of anything.

But you know, I am certain the weaker I become physically, the stronger I become inside.

I am at peace with everything, and feel strongly that this is the most amazing journey in patience, mental stamina, belief, faith, appreciation and gratitude - for everything.

I am more spiritually aware and alive than ever. It seems that great progress in these areas only comes from great challenges. Nobody (in there right mind) would want cancer. But let me tell you, it is the greatest catalyst for internal growth that I have ever experienced. Any big health issue would likely do the same.

God's plan for eternal life is eternal in measure. My bout with cancer, with eternity as the backdrop, is momentary. However, the strides in growing my soul, I feel has been accelerated to the speed of light, with monumental impact - inside me.

So when I think about how could God allow folks to suffer in this world, I also know that the momentary impact against an eternal backdrop is slight against the potential gains, which in many cases and for most of us, would likely otherwise never occur. Why should it? When we live inside comfort, the challenge to stretch is missing.

OK, this is where you will probably think I have gone mental, but in the larger scheme of things, I may well be luckier than you. The reason? If the objective we have on Earth is to prepare for eternal life in God's kingdom, than I am getting a crash course in soul building. To be honest, I like what is happening. I am stronger and better inside, than I have ever been, and I like it. So while I am beaten-up on the outside, I have gained immeasurable value inside.

Thank you God for what has been given, your guidance, and teaching. Please gently guide all my family and friends with love and care.

I will of course let you know how things turn out after I get official word on Wednesday.

Love to all!

Thursday, July 26, 2012 - Blessings Abound

It's difficult to express the depth of my gratitude for making it though a third round of cancer. Statistically I should have already died given the nature of

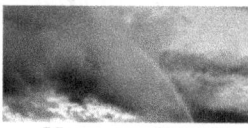

Near my House
walking the dogs

the cancer I have, based on all of the people that have gone before me. Yet, God has spared me so far.

A few weeks ago, a neighbor had a going away party for another neighbor moving to Northern California. We went over for a short visit, because chemo had me feeling poor. We met some people and had a nice time. Fast forward to last weekend. I went with the same neighbors, Dewayne and Ann our fantastic new neighbors, to a farmers market, which they had invited us to. Nearly upon arrival, the wife of a couple we had met at the party was there also buying veggies. We said hello, soon I wandered off to a stand that was selling yummy, and I mean no kidding, yummy bread.

All of a sudden, this neighbor friend, Patty, walks up to me grabs both of my hands, and pulls me aside. She stood close to me, looked directly in my eyes with an urgent expression, and said, "you need to know that all you have to do is believe Jesus has already healed you and you will be healed." She also said "I need to write the book I have been planning". It was a very powerful moment. I kissed her cheek and thanked her, and she walk away.

That was it, no other need for conversation, she left and I was left blown away - standing alone thinking about a messenger from God that was just moved by the spirit, to give me a direct communiqué. It went right through me. Wow.

So I have been thinking and praying about it a lot.

Tuesday I had a PET scan, Wednesday I learned I am in remission once again after only 3 of the 6 scheduled chemo treatments, and I know I need to write the book. I still want to finish reading the New Testament first. My thinking is that the book "Prospering with Cancer" requires a spiritual mind set, and I want to have God's word and intent correct, and therefore have much to learn biblically to do that well.

God is watching over my family in what feels like above and beyond the call of duty in many ways. I will explain more of that in the book. But it is all very amazing.

Yes I am very ill, for one thing I had to take the fourth round of chemo for mop-up reasons, but the life I do have has been made abundantly rich in blessings, from family, friends, and God's nurturing hand. This has provided great internal growth and strength, not to mention peace and happiness. I am not just saying it - I really mean exactly what I have said.

I am so grateful it makes my chest heave and my eyes water.

Thanks to you for helping me on this amazing journey. I will be getting stronger and better in the coming days and weeks.

I wish and pray for God's blessing in your life.

Today

That was my last blog entry prior to publishing the first version of this book at the end of 2012.

Since then, I have finished reading the Bible. In fact, I bought two study Bibles and read them both. Living up to the commitment, I am sitting here writing this book. There have been many lessons along the way and I have benefited greatly from them.

I have developed a nice relationship with a local Lutheran Church, and Pastor Ed Smith. Pastor Ed has been to our house several times and the conversations are lively. Pastor Ed has suggested that I have a sermon in me, which I will soon be planning.

I try to listen to Dr. John McArthur daily, which fills in lots of understanding to scripture. I also continue to read the bible in my attempts to improve knowledge.

It was impossible near the end of 2012 to predict what was going to happen. However, as I sit here now working to bring this book up to date, it is Christmas of 2013. So much more has happened in the last 17 months since I finished writing the first edition of this book. 5 months of time was spent to edit and then publish, which is why it took to the end of the 2012.

As a result, I wanted to bring it up to date.

In the following section I will pick up on the blog entries that will make the second addition of this book complete – at least up through now, which is at publication January 2014.

Round 4

Friday, October 12, 2012 - Round 4

"It takes a lot of courage to show your dreams to someone else." - Erma Bombeck

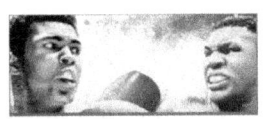

It is somehow hard to say it, I guess because I don't want to face the music, nor do I want any of you that care, to be disappointed. But I feel like cancer is back.

If so, this will be round four in this battle. While the battleground is familiar now, there is no comfort in knowing what is likely coming. On a positive note, the past skirmishes have all ended reasonably fast, so maybe, if in fact I am active, I will be in remission again by January. We shall just have to wait and see.

I have an appointment with Sam in two weeks; I suspect that I will have a PET scan in three weeks or so. We will know the story at that time.

Thursday, October 25, 2012 – It's Easy to have Faith

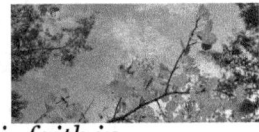

"It's easy to have faith in yourself when you're a winner, when you're number one. What you've got to have is faith in yourself when you're not a winner." -Vince Lombardi

I saw Sam! Based on my symptoms, he thinks I am active again. There is a PET scan scheduled for the 31st Halloween!

The prospect of round four has some ups and downs for me. Who in their right mind would care to have two or three months of a really bad flu. Not only is cancer a physical game, it is even more a mental game. It is really important to sincerely find the motivation to go through it again, and stay positive, and hopeful. I haven't figured out how I will do that this time, but you can be sure that I will, cause there aren't any quitters on this team folks.

On the positive side and since I saw Sam last at the end of July, two new drugs have entered the bag of tools now available.

The plan is to add the first one to the normal cocktail of chemo I currently receive, known in cancer speak as "Full Fury". It has proven to greatly enhance the effectiveness of the chemo regime. The second drug is effective at preventing it from coming back, so I will receive it as a maintenance drug.

Simply put, shrink everything that is active first, then hold it back as long as possible.

I'll let you know how things progress of course.

In the meanwhile, I haven't heard back from the publisher of my book yet. I'll let you know about that as soon as I know.

I am nearly finished scripting the presentation version of the book. I intend to record that, and post it to YouTube.

This scripture really speaks to me as a cancer patient:

*Therefore we do not lose heart. Though outwardly
we are wasting away, yet inwardly we are being
renewed day by day. For our light and momentary
troubles are achieving for us an eternal glory that
far outweighs them all. So we fix our eyes not on
what is seen, but on what is unseen. For what is seen
is temporary, but what is unseen is eternal.*
2 *Corinthians 4:16-18 (NIV)*

Sunday, October 28, 2012 – Living Next to the Tracks

**"I've learned that people will forget
what you said, people will forget
what you did, but people will never
forget how you made them feel."**

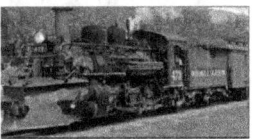

- *Maya Angelou*

*Have you ever wondered why anyone could possibly
buy a house next to a railroad track? When a train
goes by, the Earth vibrates and rumbles, you can
feel it coming before you hear it! Soon however, you
really hear it. There is nothing as loud as a train
blowing its horn. They are excruciatingly loud when
you are close. You can hear them from miles away.*

*Yet, people who do live near a train track will tell
you they don't hear the trains anymore. No matter
how loud they are, eventually the human brain can
mute them. You can hear them if you want to, but
otherwise they seem to cease behind what you are
focused on.*

The same happens at a distance. We have lived close to a track for years. Close enough that you can hear them. Sometimes in the summer, late at night I will be partially awake and hear a train coming. I will pay attention to the distinctive pattern an engineer will use in blowing the horn. I have noticed each engineer has a unique pattern of blowing the horn, like his or her personal trademark. They pass by every night, yet as I am writing this and am thinking about it, I really can't remember the last time I heard one going by. Probably months ago. I'm not purposely ignoring them, they are simply out of focus.

It seems like my chronic ordeal with cancer is having a similar phenomenon. At first the news was startling! People couldn't seem to ignore it. I suppose part of it is that cancer appears to many to be a death sentence. Now that I have beaten three rounds of it, it doesn't feel so dangerous, attention is waning.

Although it may not appear as dangerous, it really is. Kind of like living next to the train. You may not hear it, but you shouldn't play on the tracks, the stakes are way to large!

I'm entering my fourth round with cancer. The stakes are still high, the risk to my life is statistically increasing, making the game ever more dangerous. Even so, it is becoming a story that is increasingly ignored by most but the most dedicated and caring people.

I'm not complaining here, or crying out for attention. I'm just noticing this behavior and realizing how very human it is.

I thought about it a lot last night. I have decided I will continue the blog anyway for a couple of reasons. Number one, it does allow me to have a forum to keep those who wish to stay abreast of news, up to date. The second is that it helps me to crystallize my thoughts.

I really don't think what is happening reflects a lack of care. I think it has just become old news, if not an on going saga. Frankly, I don't think there are many topics that can become boring faster than aches and pains, which if anything has kept me surprised that so many people followed it at all.

For all of you that have expressed your care in one way or another in the last two years, your kind loving attention has had immeasurable value. So much so that words of thanks don't seem large enough or duly adequate. Nevertheless, thank you.

I expect a few will continue to follow regularly, others will check-in from time to time, and still others are long gone. Perhaps my presence on FaceBook is interpreted as an assurance that all is well.

If there is a surprise, and my demise happens suddenly (which it could), the blog will suddenly stop, but if there is any chance of letting you know that things have taken a critical blow, I will of course make every effort to let you know.

Bonnie asked me recently how I want things handled when I die. I told her I didn't want a funeral service. It's a long story, but I believe my body is just a shell. My spirit is what counts, and that will be with God. Therefore my body doesn't matter, and I don't need a burial or want Bonnie to incur the expense of one.

For the moment, I don't think she is planning anything. I'm just telling you this so you have a heads up to not expect a service.

I think God still has some plans for me, and if that's true, I will be around for a while. I think there is some evangelizing left to do on and for Cancer. I am putting a considerable effort into trying to fulfill that mission.

Feel free to check-in anytime you hear the whistle blow. I will always welcome you.

Thursday, November 1, 2012 - It is not the mountain we conquer but ourselves

"It is not the mountain we conquer but ourselves." - Sir Edmund Hillary

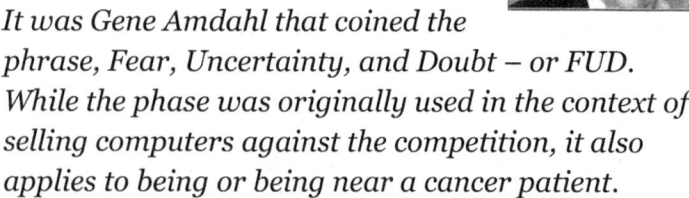

It was Gene Amdahl that coined the phrase, Fear, Uncertainty, and Doubt – or FUD. While the phase was originally used in the context of selling computers against the competition, it also applies to being or being near a cancer patient.

As you know, yesterday my read of the radiology report resulting from the PET scan was that while cancer is active in my body, it was rather small as compared to what we have seen at times in the past.

Today Dr. Sam confirmed that. Cancer is active in both my lungs and rectum, but small compared to what we have seen at times in the past.

OK, here is some disclosure, which I ordinarily don't dwell too much on, which is also a topic that we spent quite a bit of time talking about today. I have far more days where I feel really lousy than days that I feel reasonably well. Bonnie and I quizzed Sam; "why do I feel so lousy if the cancer I have is slow" and not overly active (I remind you - it is still there, just not progressing rapidly).

For the first time I think I understand this better. Whenever a disease is present in a body, part of the response of a body to mount a defense is triggered by effected cells that secrete a substance called a "Cytokine". Cytokines are small cell-signaling protein molecules that are secreted by numerous cells and are a category of signaling molecules used extensively in intercellular communication. The term "cytokine" has been used to refer to the immunomodulating agents, such as interleukins and interferons. Cytokines enhance cellular immune responses, which favor antibody responses.

So as I understand it, Cytokines interoperate with a body's autoimmune system. Adverse effects of cytokines have been linked to many disease states and conditions, ranging from major depression and Alzheimer's disease to cancer.

Over-secretion of cytokines can trigger a dangerous syndrome known as a cytokine storm. Cytokine storms were the main cause of death in the 1918 "Spanish Flu" pandemic. Cytokine storm deaths are weighted more heavily towards people with healthy immune systems, due to its ability to produce stronger immune responses, like increasing cytokine levels. Another important example of a cytokine storm is seen in acute pancreatitis.

The point of the ask Mr. Science explanation, is to understand what has been happening to me. Sam explained one cancer patient that was a train wreck on paper. He had metastatic cancer all over his body. He would walk in and claim to feel "pretty good". Things are different in my case, the amount of cancer active in my body is small, but I struggle with it. The key could be cytokines. Maybe I am having a strong cytokine reaction to cancer because I have a healthy immune system. If it was the modality of death during 1918's Spanish flu, I'm sure you can appreciate that even an elevated amount of cytokines is enough to make me fell lousy – enough at time to think I need to be in a hospital (even though I don't go).

So that explains a lot for why I feel the way I do.

In so far as where do we go from here – we are taking a little break to get through the holidays. But that doesn't mean we will do nothing. I mentioned that two new drugs have entered the market in the last 90 days. One of the new drugs is called "Stivarga", which I will begin taking immediately.

Stivarga is a pill that works by blocking several enzymes that promote cancer growth. The drug has been shown to prolong survival and slow the progression of cancer in patients whose disease has progressed after treatment with currently available therapies.

In January, I will start chemo once again to push back the cancer that is active. When that happens, I will get the second new drug, "Zaltrap." Zaltrap, like Avastin (which is a regular part of chemo therapy for me) is another angiogenesis inhibitor that inhibits the blood supply to tumors. No blood supply, no growth of the tumor. Along with one of the many genetically targeted drugs, like 5FU and Camposar, the combination is a potent approach to metastatic colo-rectal cancer (m-CRC).

Probably after about four cycles of "full-fury," now with Zaltrap, I will be finished with chemo by March. Then back to Stivarga.

So all in all, this was very good news. The reality is that I still have active cancer, but all things considered things are looking good!

I liked Sir Edmund Hillary's view. To the pessimist, still having cancer would look like bad news, but the optimist in me has me feeling excited that my chances are looking good.

What are the odds? I have about an 86%

> **Note:**
>
> Metastatic colon cancer patients have an 85% probability of dying within 5 years of contracting the disease.

probability of living for at least two years.

From where I sit, that looks terrific.

Saturday, November 17, 2012 - The Cancer Uncertainty Principle

"The best way out is always through". - Robert Frost

I am fortunate enough to be on a brand new medication from Bayer called Stivarga. It is a new class of anti-angiogenesis that hopefully will keep my cancer at bay until after the holidays, when I go back on the "Full Fury" regiment. When that happens the objective is to get me back to metabolic-remission.

None of this is a new; after all, this is my fourth bout with metastatic colo-rectal (m-CRC) cancer. I am familiar with the treatment regime, but there is no comfort in the knowledge of what is experienced.

Cancer brings an interesting challenge of uncertainty. I am naming it the Cancer Uncertainty Principle. With cancer, you just don't know your future, either in the short term, or in the long term, and therefore the things that normally are the foundation for how you find happiness - get sharply skewed.

It's not easy for many to cope with. After all, you spend your entire life either "finding yourself" or honing who you have become. You set goals, and then you measure progress. You depend on a certain set of assumptions, one of the most basic of those is your health.

After you realize what gives you joy in life, most will never question whether they will have the basic capabilities of a healthy body and mind necessary to accomplish those goals.

The removal of a fundamental requirement, your health, often removes the ability to continue to pursue dreams that have been a part of who you are, from the early years when you formed them.

This represents a large loss and possibly the most difficult challenge a person will ever face. How do you let go of who you are, and how can you find happiness when there is no certainty for either your short or long term future, thus the Cancer Uncertainty Principle.

For the last several weeks I have been feeling increasingly confident that the worst days were in back of me, at least for the foreseeable future. However, last night some of that confidence was shaken.

At about 10:30pm, I had a persistent headache that had been going on since I started Stivarga on Monday. Earlier, around 9:30 I took three ibuprofen to address the issue. I went back to bed, remembered that I should be checking my blood pressure, as this is one of the many potential side-effects of Stivarga.

My Blood Pressure was 187/116. There are many bad things that can happen to a person with a BP at that level. Brain bleeds, heart attack, kidney failure, etc. I called the on-call doctor, and shortly after headed to the local ER. Some meds for the blood pressure, pain, and a CT scan to insure my brain was OK resolved everything. But last night could

*have been a stroke, or something else equally
serious. You just don't know. You can't be certain. I
am not certain of my near-term future, nor am I
certain of my long-term future.*

*I am reminded that happiness is a personal
responsibility. It is ever more clear to me that
strong attachment to, and endless dwelling on what
I used to be, and what I used to be able to do, is the
foundation for frustration and anger. I haven't and
don't spend much time doing that. A former favorite
manager of mine, Nigel Dessau once told me, "its OK
to look back, it is impolite to stare." From the
moment I heard them I found these words to be wise
and have taken them to heart.*

*Happiness for anybody experiencing loss is about
letting go, and finding the joy in the things that are
realistically around you right now. I feel certain
that faith is also a critical ingredient for happiness.
If cancer is the uncertainty principle, it is only so
because of an unrealistic perspective and attitude.*

*My life has changed. It will never be the same as it
was. I am not able to do the things I used to do. I
don't know if I will be in an ER tonight. I don't know
if I will be alive in a year. But I do know that as I
am writing this, I am listening to some beautiful
music. Bonnie and I cooked breakfast together this
morning. My dogs had a bath yesterday. They smell
wonderful, and are soft and pretty. I will be going
to a church service tomorrow, and then have a
member lunch there tomorrow. I am still working
on formatting edits for my book to get it accepted by
Amazon, and that is nearly done. I just bought a*

Nikon GPS for my camera to tag pictures with location data.

Three friends have called to check on me just this morning, because they care. Thanksgiving is next week, and I will have time to be with some of my family, no matter how I feel.

Cancer causes uncertainty, for things in the past. Cancer creates uncertainty for how much runway is left for your future. But I am in control of what happens in between. I love and am grateful to God, family and friends, for the joy they bring. I have faith in all of them to care for me, and to provide the motivation to continue to live and to find joy and happiness everyday.

Cancer has taken my past, but I am building my future, finding joy, and am grateful that I am still alive - because the joy I find in this life is rewarding and worth the trouble.

Thanks to my medical team for catching me this week.

May God's blessing bring you happiness and joy everyday.

Friday, December 7, 2012 - The Thorn in my Life

"God uses the problem to make us aware of our need, so that we look up instead of looking inward in our own strength." – Dr. David Jeremiah

I started the new drug Stivarga at one quarter strength from the last time, again on Tuesday, and I was ill by evening. I don't think I get along with this drug. The headache was bad enough that it took morphine to tolerate it – ouch! Of course all of the other chemo symptoms were there as well.

The difference between what I normally get for chemo symptoms and this drug - is the additional symptoms of a crushing headache and elevated blood pressure. Whatever, I took it as a second attempt Tuesday and Wednesday, and quit again Thursday morning. This stuff is just too much, or my body doesn't handle it well. I am finished with it.

So that means, I start the infusion variety chemo again January 2nd, joy.

That brings us too the thorn part. While there is no doubt that cancer, chemo, and illness is down right nasty, through the struggle it has once again reminded me that as I weaken under the load of physical strain imposed by the oppressive weight of cancer, it somehow induces me to look out and up for thanks.

From my old self, it doesn't seem logical to do this. From my spiritually awakened new self, it seems to be the only thing that makes sense. I can lay awake at night caused by one issue or another, and I think through a conversation with God cataloging all of the things that have happened in my life, or are currently happening - that I am grateful for. Things that seem silly in some ways, as I think about them while writing this. But when it comes down to the core measure of the things that are important in life, as I have written so often about, they really are the only and true measure of value. It is easy for so many to question the existence of a living God. It is also easy for all that have found faith to know, that every comfort, from the small and overlooked, to the most major and consequential, are a gift. These gifts are always there, but so often unobserved by the blindness of worldly involvement.

For some when the thorn arrives, it only inspires resentment or worse, which can be focused in all sorts of directions. For some it is internal, for others it is a way to lash out externally.

How lucky are the ones that see beyond the thorn, to know that the lesson is difficult, but the awakening generated - is beyond calculation in value, because it is measured on an eternal scale.

Really I am not a skipping through the daisies type of person. Yet it is true that I am positive generally. But the thorn given to me, has taken me to places I have never been before, nor would I have likely achieved without.

I pray that if and when your thorn arrives, you have the perspective to gain the value for what is offered.

On a positive ending note, "Prospering with Cancer" is published in both print and Kindle!

Hooray! When I hold the finished book in my hand, I don't feel a sense of accomplishment as some PhD investigative study, as a result of the modesty in page count. However, I equally do feel what the book lacks in size, it makes up for in spirit. Even when I was writing it, I felt it couldn't be a novel in size, because the audience most likely to read it would not have the focus or energy for that.

I also feel the book was required to pay forward the loving support of so many, and hope it offers a context in which people can look at their thorn, and develop the vision for their lessons of joy.

God Bless all of you.

Monday, December 10, 2012 - Cancer's Fear: Coward or Courageous?

"Fear makes men forget, and skill - which cannot fight, is useless." — Phormio of Athens

People have been going to battle for thousands of years. Warfare has always been a human endeavor, whether it is carrying a weapon on a battlefield, walking in to see a medical team or even sitting down in an infusion center, the stakes are as extreme. Maslow's law prioritizes the experience as the number one issue on anybody's mind; survival.

[1]Sir John Desmond Patrick Keegan was a British military historian, lecturer, writer and journalist. In his study of Agincourt, Waterloo, and the Somme, he notes, "What battles have in common is human: the behavior of men struggling to reconcile their instinct for self preservation, their sense of honor and the achievement of some aim over which other men are ready to kill them.

For the many battling cancer, the effect is similar, with one exception. For us, the battle is with no human being, it is with a formidable adversary whose aim is also to kill us. Many never see the enemy, but we know it is there. We observe the damage from the battle. We feel the wounds from battle. We feel the fear of battle. We watch our families and friends suffer with their fears and their psychological wounds caused by our battle. In

---

[1] Military Citations: (Major Gregory A. Daddis, 2004)

military terms it is known as collateral damage and it is devastating. Not only to those that suffer it, but perhaps even more by us, the cancer soldiers, who may have an added sense of guilt resulting from the harm to others, the people that are gallantly and courageously offering their love and support. An offering that becomes critically important to the cancer soldier, in harnessing and controlling our fears.

People have been struggling to deal with battle fears from the beginning of time.

Greek moralist Plutarch relates how the Roman general Aemilius Paulus, viewing the Greek formations at the battle of Pydna in 168, "considered the formidable appearance of their front, bristling with arms, and was taken with both fear and alarm; nothing he had ever seen before was its equal."

A similar reaction occurred at the battle of Waterloo in 1815 when French General Jean Baptiste d'Erlon's attacking corps met the British infantry's steady fire. Of interest is that the soldiers in the least immediate danger bolted first. One French officer said, "As we approached at a moderate pace the fronts and flanks began to turn their backs inwards (to run away); the rear of the columns had already begun to run away."

It is certain that cancer patients and caregivers have also faced fears that resonate with their very core instinct to survive. But unlike the battlefield soldier, the cancer soldier has no place to run. With cancer, running from fear is only an accelerated approach to suffering and death. There is really only one sensible response, and that is to stay in formation, and face the cancer enemy.

For historical military leaders to make an impression on frightened soldiers during the era of close order formations, was much simpler than it is today. Then, soldiers standing shoulder to shoulder gained strength from close physical contact and from their officers, whose definition of courage required them to face enemy fire unperturbed, much as a cancer soldier must today. One Union soldier advancing on Fort Donelson, Tennessee, in 1862 gained courage from General C.F. Smith, who rode calmly among a hail of Confederate mini-balls: "I was scared to death, but I saw the old man's white mustache over his shoulder, and went on." A cancer soldier doesn't have a mounted General with saber in hand to rally us, but we do have incredible medical teams that serve similar functions to rally and lead our personal battle.

For the military soldier, leadership is not a choice. You either have great leadership that understands the dynamics of how leaders guide training and practice that creates a psychological framework from which you can manage your fear in the chaos of battle, or you are on your own. The cancer soldier's fortune is better, you can choose the medical team that inspires and builds confidence in you, allowing you to make treatment decisions. Wasting time on the cancer battlefield is dangerous; the cancer soldier must aggressively engage the weapons of cancer, and trust the medical team to lead the charge.

Historian Joanna Burke observes, "The longer the feelings of isolation and confusion of battle lasted, the less likely it was that anyone would act aggressively." Cancer soldiers all start the battle feeling alone, but in stark contrast to the warfighter, cancer solders have a choice. If we have the framework to understand how critically important our medical leadership is and how they must perform, then we have the ability to measure them, and choose carefully and rapidly who we will entrust to rally the necessary and correct resources on our behalf. We will know if they have the ability to train us to give us the confidence we need for our battles without fears.

Individual factors can stimulate fear just as easily as the operational environment can. In his memoir, William Manchester recalls his fright while fighting in the Pacific during World War II. He felt paralyzed with fear one night in part because of his active imagination: "A fresh fear was creeping over my mind, quietly, stealthily, imperceptibly. I sat up; my muscles rippling with suppressed panic."

In the battle of cancer, wondering if a malignancy will metastasize can be equally troubling. While there is no sudden rush through the jungle from war fighters, cancer is still frightening, and maybe more so. With cancer, you don't have the luxury of seeing an enemy approaching, you don't have a way to assess the level of the threat and you can't shoot at it. With cancer, you may have already taken a bullet, and may not really be aware of it until your next diagnostic scan, leaving lots of time to imagine how bad things may become from something that can be as deadly as a bullet.

U.S. Marine Corps Lieutenant Philip Caputo was equally stunned by the muddled, unforgiving environment of Vietnam. Caputo found that men with lively imaginations are prey to fears: "A man needs many things in war, but a strong imagination is not one of them. In Vietnam, the best soldiers were usually unimaginative men who did not feel afraid until there was obvious reason."

Added to the difficulty of assessing fear-producing elements in battle is the fact that individuals have varying capacities to deal with the stresses of combat. Within those individuals, and even units, fear and courage are often an unpredictable phenomena. Soldiers who stand fast on one day might break under the strain of battle the next. In cancer you need faith and to not over-think the problem as well. Doctors are trained and skillful at predicting and managing the risks. A cancer soldier must choose the right team, but then you must have faith in them, realizing that they too have better days than others.

Even with great leadership, any contemporary military or cancer battlefield can produce the anxiety of being alone. Like the warfighter in a foxhole, the cancer soldier eventually and frequently is alone with their imagination. Reassurance from nearby friends, which strengthens resolve against the enemy and his weaponry, withers when friendly sights and sounds are absent. In my battle with cancer, I have known from the beginning how valuable the support from my family and friends have been, but until recently I was never able to put my finger on exactly why. The answer was too simple. Cancer spawning fear is rooted in uncertainty, suffering and ultimately the possibility of death. Supporting medical teams, family and friends act to provide compassion that translates ultimately to courage.

S.L.A. Marshall offers his soundest arguments in Men Against Fire: The Problem of Battle Command in Future War, where he discusses tactical cohesion and why men fight. Marshall asserts that personal honor is a powerful motivator in battle and that soldiers rarely aspire to unworthiness. Still, either through physical or social isolation, men fall prey to their fears and provide no combat value to the organization.

Underscoring the importance of unity, Marshall emphasizes the "inherent unwillingness of the soldier to risk danger on behalf of men with whom he has no social identity." I assert that the social identity feeds a sense of self worth. When people are expressing their affection and care, the feeling of self worth is elevated, providing a measure of value used to increase the will to fight.

The battle with cancer is the same as a war fighters'. Constant contact with supporters address a sense of isolation, it also develops a sense of worthiness and honor. That sets the stage for steeling up to engage the battle without fear or cowardice.

An observer often sees taking the cancer battle head-on as brave and courageous. Really it is neither. How often have we seen people in uniform, with what appears to be no personal fear, jump into some life saving situation to save the day? Their courage in the end is really the execution of a large amount of well-rehearsed training. When stress is high, and urgency is exigent, people revert to what they are trained to do. They are not paralyzed with fear, they are cognitively evaluating options, and then suddenly and deftly they execute. When interviewed afterward, they always say, "I was just doing my job." Which is appealing because we still think they are heroes and have courage.

The battle with cancer is similar. A cancer soldier has no place to run even if they were so inclined. The only option is to stand your ground and take it on.

The medical team provides the leadership, training, resource management, and steady hand we depend on. Family and friends are motivators, preventing us from feeling alone, and making us aware that our measure of personal honor is set from not wanting to let those that love us down.

Preparing soldiers to deal with fear is indispensable for maintaining cancer combat readiness. In our society, the people we consider courageous are a special few. They are people we respect, admire and aspire to be. One never really knows how you will respond to difficult circumstances when the stakes are as high as suffering and death. But one thing is certain, without a medical team to provide expert leadership and care, without friends and family to provide loving and caring support, the likelihood of surviving a bravely fought battle is greatly reduced.

I am not so callous that I can write this without the Lords share. All of the psychological drivers are true and important. After all, most doctors will tell you that the single strongest determining factor in your recovery is a strong positive mental attitude, and everything above address that.

Nevertheless, God's will supersedes all of it. The plan is either a thorn that drives learning, awakening and spiritual development, or an exit strategy to deliver you back into the hands of God. That too is not something that is revealed to you, so you must act as if your life depends on it, because it does.

To the caregivers, family and friends, your contribution saves lives, which you will feel as a reward, and God will celebrate.

To all the war-fighters and cancer soldiers, have faith, and be courageous, it makes a difference. God's blessings.

Monday, December 31, 2012 - Fall
seven times, stand up eight

七転び八起き

"Fall down seven times, stand up eight"

Japanese Proverb

Cancer is back, and making itself known. My last chemo treatment happened July 25th, 2012. So, I have had a fair stretch off from the last treatment. I have known that round four of the cancer was active and growing for a few months, but avoiding the inevitable. Sort of. I did take a new drug, Stivarga, but I didn't tolerate it at all. It was so bad I had to stop. So, while there was a chance of preventing the need for more infusion, it just didn't work out.

Where would your mind be? On the negative side, getting mentally up for the punishment ahead is never easy, for me, or anyone. Therefore, and naturally, I would just as soon skip the next few months. Nothing realistic about that however. Wednesday will be here soon, and I must face the music with chin and attitude up and intentions true.

As I wrote in the last blog, it's not courage, it's simply what has to happen, and just like before I will get through this again.

It's really important to have a prize to keep your eye on. For me, I know chemo will end no later than the end of February when I will be at the bottom of my strength and endurance. In March I will be getting stronger, and in April, we will bring the motor home out of cold storage. We will likely head for California where I expect to photograph the redwoods and the coast. Maybe even camp in Yosemite again, which is a great place for photography.

I wonder how many more times I will have to do this before the medicine will no longer work. Hopefully I will last long enough for a new medical option to emerge that can more than just slow it, but actually stop it. We shall see.

In the meanwhile, I am working to put round four in the history books, so I can stand up to prepare to savor the life I share with family and friends.

I have many things to work on to keep mentally engaged, but I think I will add reading the bible over again to the list.

There are so any blessings in my life I am so grateful for.

I hope your blessings meet all of your needs as well.

Wednesday, January 2, 2013 - Happy New Year, and Hopes for a Great 2013

We have all had challenges in 2013. I keep thinking about the thought that what doesn't kill you makes you stronger. I certainly have benefited from spiritual and human awakening that was spawned by my brush with mortality.

Cancer is an ugly beast, but what can happen in your soul is fortunate, and I for one am grateful for that. Cancer has taught me to be a better person, and to appreciate the good in others, as well as tolerance for what is not so good.

In the end, I believe that is what God wanted all along. Now I just have to try to continue to refine both.

I wish all of you nothing but the best in 2013. While ideal health may not be your best achievement, I pray that you see the gifts and appreciate all of the other gifts that are there for you.

Best wishes to all, and God's very best blessings!

Happy New Year!

Wednesday, January 9, 2013 - Cancer's Loving Light

"Not all of us can do great things.
But we can do small things with
great love." - Mother Teresa

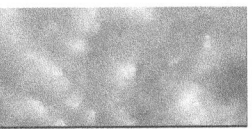

Many people who don't have cancer seem to think
that to have cancer is to be stuck in endless longing
of existing in a slow motion movie of a perfectly
toned body running on a beach exuding the most
vibrant body of strength, stamina and health.

Not to be contrary, but that isn't what I wish for.
For me, I tend to wish to enjoy each day as the
blessing it is, and wish that all my friends could
understand the joy that family, friends, and faith
have and continue to bring me.

Starring at mortality has been the catalyst to
understand this. I am afraid that wishing for only
health, is a form of hanging onto something I have
lost, at the possible expense of missing all of what I
have gained and what is still possible too.

Health is important to be sure, but I believe what I
have found is more important and is eternal. I'm
really not sure I would trade it now.

Before you think I am crazy, I must tell you that I
have talked with some pretty brave and beautiful
souls. As an example, in the infusion center just this
week I sat next to a couple that have been married
for nearly fifty years. The gentleman was getting

infused and was looking like he was taking the full brunt of it. We were there for some six hours together. He was in and out of sleep. When he did feel like it, we spoke. We talked about the nice meal they severed us, a baked Salmon. We talked about how amazing and loving the people are that are taking care of us. What a wonderful life he and his bride have had together. They worked and played together for a lifetime. The places we have been, the great people on the planet.

He asked about my cancer, I briefly told him. He told me about his. A very aggressive cancer, which is now in most of his organs. He has only known about his cancer for a few months. He didn't moan about anything really. He didn't lament about his illness or his chances. He focused on things that are bright and beautiful, and wished me well.

There are lots of facets to life, and health is a big one. But for myself and many others along the cancer journey, the world doesn't end with the diagnosis. Life is more of a cumulative event to me. Certainly a large part of who I am is defined by all of the things, good and bad, I have done in sickness and in health. But as health has become an issue, I certainly don't find that I have lost the ability to grow, contribute, and to find joy. However, it has changed to be sure.

That seems to be the point of happiness in general. The only thing in life you can truly count on is change. The easier you shift with change, and remain true to who you really are, the more easily you adapt and continue happily down life's challenges and offerings.

It is a lesson in humility to witness the humility of so many people that have gone over the cancer speed bump, and continue to live in joy.

It is another data point that makes me believe in the power of God's love shining through, may you all experience it abundantly.

Saturday, January 26, 2013 - You Can't Ring Out with Cancer

If you read my blog post "Cancer's Fear – Coward or Courageous", you know that I see a direct parallel with the cancer fighter and a war fighter. I have realized a few interesting differences as well.

I have always admired the training the US military provides for today's soldiers. Our military takes young men and women from the homes they grew up in, and molds them rapidly with skills, physical conditioning, discipline and strength. They also learn to have courage, commitment, and honor. One of the major factors to the success of the US military is their ability to also help soldiers learn that they can do more than they previously believed possible - by themselves.

US Military Special Forces are particularly good at this. We all know the capabilities of US Rangers, Marine Special Operations, Air Force Pararescue, and Navy Seal teams are legendary. They endure ridiculous amounts of pain, physical discomforts (like freezing cold or hot conditions), hunger, stress, sleep deprivation and yet they efficiently keep going to accomplish their assigned mission against overwhelming odds. In training people to have these capabilities, cadets are put through punishing treatment as a part of their conditioning. This must be done so that the cadet can learn how far they can go, and how much they can tolerate and still function as an individual and in a unit.

*There is no training in the world that is more
demanding and difficult than the US Navy Seal
Basic Underwater Demolition and Seal training,
known as BUD/s. Roughly 80% of the elite sailors
that are selected for BUD/s training washout! The
hardest part varies and depends on the individual.
Some people can't take the physical training, or
some part of it. For some, swimming is easy and
running is hard, for others the swimming is the hard
part. Some can't take the stress. Some can't take the
intensity. Some can't take the pain. Some can't take
the cold water off the coast of San Diego where they
train and are constantly wet. Maybe the worst part
is what they call Hell Week. 24 hours a day for a
whole week, they dish out punishing training, and
all of it while they are seriously sleep deprived.*

*Seals are not made, they are found. They emerge
out of the rigors of intense training where they have
survived punishment others could not. Yet nobody is
told to leave unless they are just physically unable to
keep up. Otherwise, each person that fails the
program simply makes a personal decision that they
have had enough. When they reach that point and
are ready to quit, they fall out of line, and go ring a
nearby brass bell. When they do, they are
considered Dropped On Request or DOR. There is
no shame in it. The Navy only wants the ones that
can operate in adverse conditions that few on this
planet can. They have to have mental toughness and
an unwavering commitment to never give up.
Giving up for them is just not an option.*

For those that can't take the punishment, ringing that bell means warmth, a bed, rest, food, and things becoming far more comfortable in a hurry.

But I wonder, if they knew that ringing the bell meant they would die, how many more of them would instead reach a little deeper, go a little further, and make it through the training to not just survive, but to be able to claim a victory they didn't expect they could achieve?

I think that is what it is like to have cancer. For me it has been like being stuck in a very physically demanding, stressful, uncomfortable at times bordering on suffering situation. For the cancer fighter, ringing the bell means you have decided it is time to die. People certainly do get there mentally and physically. There is a limit to what a human is able to or willing to endure. The tolerance threshold is individually decided and derived, but some people do decide to die. I don't see that as a disgrace. But I do believe, that the preponderance of cancer survivor's have gone beyond what most people realize in what a cancer fighter has been able to tolerate, and yet – they often still come up smiling.

I am nowhere close to any of that. I am just realizing that my appreciation continues to grow for the cancer fighters that stand up to the punishment of cancer so courageously. Cancer survivors feel like they have accomplished something, and in part, their determination is a part of it. It is just raw determination to gut it out because quitting is not an option. My pride in these people continues to grow.

I wish there were a way to award military style medals for bravery.

If there were a way, everybody would get a purple heart for being wounded in action while engaging the cancer enemy. Medals would be awarded for valor and conferred to individuals who distinguished themselves in the cancer battle. Recipients would include those that have courageously acted beyond the call of duty for both the good of themselves, and the good of their family and friends.

Maybe the Medal of Honor could be awarded to those that make great contributions to cancer research, the Distinguished Service Cross for extreme gallantry while battling cancer, the Silver Star for gallantry, and the Bronze star could be awarded for acts of heroism and merit. All of the medals could represent valor and intensity for the fight with cancer.

The human spirit's will to survive difficult conditions is massively inspiring. The noble among us don't know they were born with a level of gallantry and courage that awes and inspires others when it rises to overwhelm difficult odds. But when we are lucky enough to observe it in people we are close to it is humbling to our very soul.

God Bless the courageous and gallant souls, you give us all something to aspire to.

Thursday, January 31, 2013 - "Patience - the gift of being able to see past the emotion."

I have been on this cancer journey for 2 years and 6 months. I am still alive, and I have beaten the statistical odds. I just had a chemo blast yesterday, and in fact the chemo pump is on

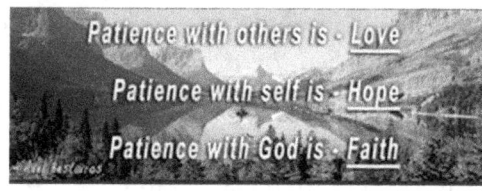

while I am writing this. I feel chemo ill. Headache, nausea, achy, fatigue. I woke up at 3:30 and got up at 4am. I'm tired. All of this is normal and to be expected.

I want to feel healthy enough to go ride my bike and build strength and stamina, but can't because I am to weak, and it would just make me more ill. It would in fact only result in getting physically punished.

I can think reasonably well for half a day, and am engaged in various mental pursuits including acting as an advisor in the IT industry. When I have sat here long enough I begin to get ill and must stop. Usually by noon. Going out to dinner with someone is impossible without being punished. Usually I will be in bed by 6pm.

Cancer causes all of this, treatment just makes it far worse.

I continue to think that cancer is a test of patience. I decided I would write a blog post this morning and found the quotes above. The quote I Photoshopped

*into the picture hit what I feel- square on the head.
Since beginning the cancer journey, those
realizations have best and most succinctly epitomize
what I have learned and what I am grateful for.*

*I have learned also that these lessons of discovery
are better served in the cancer community. The
reads on my personal blog is a trickle now, for each
of my posts. The people that were reading it on my
web-site, have largely lost the interest in what
appears to be an ongoing saga with no end. Which
by the way, I understand. However while the story
hasn't changed in any major way that grasps the
interest of a large following of people that don't have
cancer, it nevertheless occupies my thoughts and
activities or lack of them.*

*The people that do find the week-to-week musing
interesting are the cancer communities. I post on
Blog for a Cure.*

*The most important thing to me, is to keep friends
that want to know what is happening up to date,
and to offer cancer survivors a context that is
positive, to help them through the mental challenges
that are so troubling, based on all of the issues
caused by the disease. Cancer patients loose many
things, but without a doubt there are things to be
deeply grateful for, and joyful over. I am living my
life from joy regardless of what is taken from me.
But it is a test of patience! I hope I can help others to
see how that is done. For some, it may be difficult to
find, but for all that do find joy, the benefits are
without measure.*

That is what I like about Stand Up 2 Cancer (SU2C), they look for ways to improve the lives of cancer survivors, and they get involved in doing that in benevolent ways. I can stand behind and up for that.

May Gods blessing be abundant for you.

Monday, February 11, 2013 - Someone you Love is Dying, Now What?

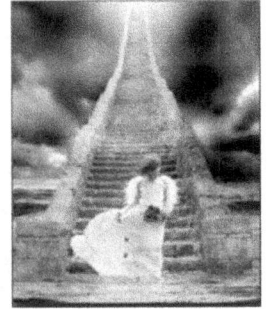

Revelation 21:4 "God will take away all their tears. There will be no more death or sorrow or crying or pain. All the old things have passed away."

There is no "one size fits all" answer to this question. There are so many people that are all different in so many ways. We have all had different lives, educations, jobs, family, friends, and colleagues. Everyone knows we are all different.

But after you get past all of the veneer described above, what's left. When each person is alone with their thoughts and are facing mortality, then how different are we. As a "terminal" patient, I have watched to see how others are dealing with it. I have to say the vast majority of people I have watched are resolved and happy overall.

Of course there is sadness for everybody. We love lots of people, and knowing that someone we love is soon going to be gone accelerates our passion and care for that individual. You could miss the opportunity to really let that person know how much they mean to you, and you don't want that to happen.

I can tell you that within the first three months of being told I had terminal cancer I heard "I love you" more than I think I had heard it in my entire life.

Who knew? Who knew so many people felt a need to let me know?

You know what you need? But have you really thought about what your dying loved one needs or wants?

I think it is fair to say that I have seen two types of people facing death. In one small camp there are people that are really angry. They don't want to die, they are angry about what they perceive they are loosing and they can't accept it, or anything else. They are mad at people and they are mad at God. Wow!

For these people, it is really hard to share your love. They are so focused on their own loss, there isn't much room to bring them comfort and joy. But of course you have to try. Being there for them may even be an annoyance because it interrupts them from feeling sorry for themselves and focusing on their own anger. You need to tell them you love them anyway of course and hope it resonates. Really what else can you do?

Just like any other issue that causes people to disengage, there is a certain amount of self-responsibility involved in your own balanced well-being. If a person is angry about dying, they are either going to resolve their feeling and communicate what is really important to them, which is the better outcome, or they are going to die angry with a sense of bring robbed.

I think the above scenario is a small percentage. I think most people become acutely aware of how precious the rest of their life is, and how precious all the people that are in their life are to them. They more or less are filled with love and want to express that love. They want people to know what they mean to them and how important they have been to their life. They want to thank others for their kindness and contributions. They want other to feel how much they appreciate all of these things.

So the question is, what does that near death person want? Probably what you are already giving them – love. But look, nothing is more easy, nor probably more valuable, than just being there and letting them know you care. Let them know that they have also made a difference to your life. Tell them why. In the end, I think that most people realize that what matters has nothing to do with any material point of prestige. It has everything to do with two things, love for God and humanity. Those are the two things that count; you take with you and have left behind.

So what messages will matter to a person that is dying? Things that have to do with love. Obviously sending a get-well card is senseless. Sending a card that expresses how that person has made a difference in your life does. A message that reassures a person of God's love and the kingdom that waits will also matter. Expressing the joy of a heavenly re-united family matters. All of these things are true and to the point.

A dying person may be concerned for the support they can no longer provide to a family or person.

Letting them know you are OK, and will manage to stay OK will help to relive them of potential guilt.

Letting them know it is OK to return to God, helps to reduce potential fear they may have of passing.

Loving them as they pass is maybe one of the more generous things any human can offer another. You can be sad to lose a person, but a sense of celebration should be felt for the glory of being in God, heaven, and waiting family members presence. You can even express your waiting anticipation for joining them too.

This may seem morose to you. If so I would suggest that our culture is not very well trained in knowing what the right things are to do and say, which leaves us feeling awkward, which leaves many silent or absent. Perhaps more than at any other point in the human experience, dying is the time that a person most needs the love their circle of family, friends, and colleagues can offer.

It's the grand finale of everything that person has done. It is the time to celebrate shared experiences and the bonds of friendship and love that will never expire. It is the most significant time in a persons life to let them know they have mattered in your life and why.

It is a time for generosity of human compassion to be shared and the value that life has offered to be savored. It is a time to say farewell to those that are returning to God's kingdom, and to let them know that you are right with it.

More than anything it is about love. Share your love - it's what matters.

Wednesday, February 13, 2013 - Near Completion

We saw Sam yesterday. Based on clinical presentation, it appears that I am nearly ready to close the books on round four of cancer. I 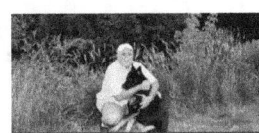 *have chemo today. But next Tuesday I am scheduled for a PET scan. I will get the official results on Wednesday, when I expect I will be in remission. Unfortunately, I will have one more round of chemo the same day - no matter what.*

So one more chapter of cancer and chemo will be done. What gives me pause, is to think of how many more times will I get through it before the chemo stops working.

Sam is opening his books to start searching for clinical trials that may be useful to me. There are a couple of new things that may help.

So – all in all I have gotten though this without much fan-fare. One more to go, two weeks of wondering, and this one is history.

Sunday, February 17, 2013 - Waiting for Destiny

"It is not in the stars to hold our destiny but in ourselves."
— *William Shakespeare*

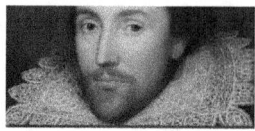

Even though my favorite oncologist, and friend Sam told me in the beginning of the cancer journey that I am terminal, I have continued to live and fight the battle as if I am going to beat cancer. The statistical reality is that I will not, and I know that, unless there is some miracle breakthrough.

It creates an odd mental conundrum. In some regards, I play life as if it will go on, business as usual, with no more or less risk that what you have in your life. I am engaged in cancer awareness efforts through blogging, and even Twitter now, acting as an advisory on an advisory board for high tech companies, planning this summer in the motor home, and considering new techniques and scenic settings for photography. All of that amounts to 'living life' type of thoughts. It's not phony either. I am mentally, emotionally, and spiritually happy.

I am near closing the books on round 4 of cancer. The accomplishment of winning four rounds of cancer has not come without a price. I have lost health and strength in many measures. I am physically unable to do many things I used to never give a thought to. Like mowing the yard as an example, or even just carrying heavy things around. I can get up and have a pretty productive brain for half a day before becoming fatigued and being forced to lie down or suffer the physical penalty. All of that is worse while on chemo, because chemo for me, and at this point, is worse than the disease. Round 5 of cancer is out on the horizon somewhere lurking and waiting to strike again.

So what do I have to look forward to? The reality is that at some point my body will reject the healing benefits of chemo, cancer runs amuck, and I become increasingly dysfunctional, sick and then die. Joy (with sarcasm).

I had a bit of a silent and subtle wake up call this week when I saw Sam. He wants to start looking at all available clinical trials available for a person in my spot. He wants to do that ahead of the time that we run out of options on chemo working, which is the good news. The bad news is that he must realize that as far past the statistical boundary as I am, that cancer is getting closer to catching up with and overwhelming me regardless of how positive I fight the battle. After all, I am 2.5 years into an original estimate of living .5 to 1.5 years.

I have a feeling that either we find some new approach or I will become as mortal as everyone else in this situation, and truly, at some point the disease will overwhelm me. Now, nobody can say with any degree of certainty when that happens, and truly I could last another five years as an example.

But the longer I go, the more pressure there is to find something that will stop the disease besides the standard approach I am on now. There are plenty of new and exciting things that are going on. One involves a virus that has two genetically engineered missing proteins. One prevents it from multiplying and renders the virus inert to normal cells. Which is good because the virus is a variant of smallpox known as vaccinia. However, when that virus "sees" a "hospitable" malignant cancer cell, BAM, it wakes up by borrowing proteins that are available only in the cancer cell, which trigger a full scale and aggressive autoimmune attack to kill cancer. For the group treated, they would have expected a survival rate of 4 or 5 months, yet some that were treated lived a year or two longer! Notice it didn't "cure" them. But it gave them a lot more runway.

For many including me, I am happy with a longer life just to continue to enjoy the joy of family, friends, colleagues and so many of God's blessings. But I could also see that if the time comes when the disease has robbed me of the joy of living that I would be ready to pass on. Purely a non-emotional and intellectual perspective. Easy to say now, it may be difficult to say or think later.

I am grateful for the blessings received in vast amounts after developing cancer. I feel fortunate that I realized the many blessing around me, were worth fighting and living for, at the very same time many other things were being taken away. Oddly, the arrival rate of new blessings seems to outpace the loss rate of things that are now gone.

I am also certain that a positive frame of mind is crucial to happiness and survival that goes beyond the statistical boundaries.

New to my thinking is that there is an end game to think about. I need to review all that is important to me, and make sure I am spending my time on the things that count, and that bring joy to myself and others. Prioritization has never been more important with an out come that is so pivotal. As humans we cannot have a perfectly executed life bringing the most perfect outcome.

The question is, how much can you improve on the execution of who you are in the time that you have left? Can you move the needle forward? Can you make a difference in areas that count? Have you thought about what really matters? That is my task.

I want to contribute more to help others, always the pressure of so much to do, with so little time.

Wednesday, February 20, 2013 - God Bless the Medical Teams

"We must find time to stop and thank the people who make a difference in our lives." - John F Kennedy

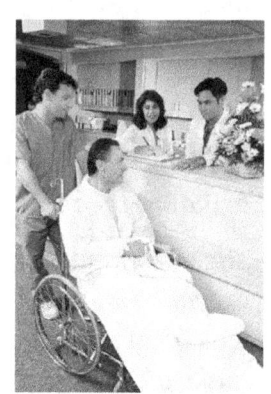

If you have cancer you know how mentally consuming it can be. Of course it is more than just about you. There is a large circle impacted of family, friends, and colleagues. I have been in this battle for 2.5 years, though four bouts of cancer and I have given this a lot of thought.

Just when I thought I had done a good job of thinking that I was including everyone around me, in considering how my cancer impacts them, I realized how remiss I have been.

My medical team has of course been engaged, thoughtful and competent at taking care of me. However I was dumbstruck this week when I realized that I have only considered what goes on with them professionally. I have completely ignored the human impact they must endure. I continue to amaze myself at how stupid I can be. Of course, the nurses and Sam, my oncologist and team hug me and are concerned, I know that. What I don't know is how they do it.

How can they continue to treat, and care for me and others, and not be emotionally involved? And since they are emotionally involved as humans, how do they continue to motivate themselves for a best effort, when they know that some they will treat, simply won't (likely) make it? How do they dig up the professionalism and personal courage to know they are stepping onto an emotional land mine? These people are not the exception, they are overwhelmingly the rule. You can't pay them to have the compassion and care they do, because money doesn't buy that.

This comes from souls that are good and exemplify the finest qualities that can be found in humanity. Their dedicated resolve to aid, takes the command to "love thy neighbor" to a whole different level. Many of us that battle the disease are grateful beyond what simple words can convey for the time you give us to do what matters, be with our family and friends, and deepen our faith in God.

Your contribution is a gift we receive of heavenly worthiness and there is no way to pay it back in equal measure. You are our angels, and only God has a position great enough to adequately thank you.

I am amazed and humbled by your dedication of contribution that is so meaningful. I'm not sure any of us patients really understand the many sacrifices you so willingly give, that allow us to live.

I also don't understand how you deal with the human drama you must so often be exposed too. Thank God you do somehow know how to cope with that, and you happily practice your craft and good deeds.

Not only do you practice the trade you have chosen and worked so hard to be excellent in, you have transcended the obligations of - just a job.

You have shown tender concern and care that comes from your heart and is directed to all of us that battle a disease that robs us of the life we knew, and in some cases life itself.

Your teams work with a sense of urgency to find treatments that help us to heal. But that's not good enough.

Your teams have set the goal to eradicate the relentless progress of this retched disease. Many of us owe the life we have today to your efforts. What we owe you is larger than money, we owe you a debt of gratitude and thanks.

While it is nowhere close to commensurate, I just want thank you. Your care adds positive value, to what can be a very difficult personal challenge that so many of us face.

God bless all of you.

Monday, February 25, 2013 - Hospital Surprise

"What seems to us as bitter trials are often blessings in disguise."
- Oscar Wilde

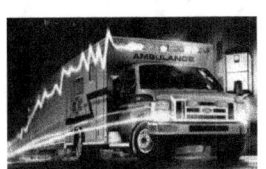

I thought I should do an update on the events from last week.

Tuesday Bonnie and I were walking the dogs when I mentioned, gee – nothing has happened this chemo cycle. As in - the usual hospital ER visit from some bizarre unexpected event.

Wednesday morning I got up at 4am to write the blog on thanks to the medical teams. Around 7am had breakfast with Bonnie. Then I started feeling cold. So I went over and sat in front of the fireplace for a while. Then I started shivering. Oh, been there before, not a good sign. I hurried into the bedroom, got under the covers and turned the electric blanket to 12. The shivers turned to rigor where there is an exaggerated amount of shaking usually associated with a high fever. It occurs because cytokines are released as part of an immune response and increases the set point for body temperature in your brain. The increased set point causes your body temperature to rise, but also makes you feel cold until the new set point is reached. The shivering in a physiological attempt to increase body temperature to the new set point.

Because I didn't know what else was happening, or the potential impact, it was time to call 911.

Minutes later, the big red truck and ambulance were parked in front of the house. A squad of paramedics was in my bedroom playing twenty questions, and doing vitals. Blood pressure was 200/140. Time to go to the hospital. Rigor ceased in the ambulance.

In ER they took blood to culture it to see if there was an infection, and more blood to do a full blood panel.

An hour later they had identified the issue. My white blood cell count was significantly below the minimum low, same for red, and I had an unidentified infection. Of course there was a small fever too. That's when I was admitted and was told I would be there for two to three days minimum.

Treatment was an antibiotic infusion that was running continuously. I was sick, and had a crushing migraine headache. The day and night were pretty rough. However, around 4am I started to feel better. They took blood around 6am for more lab work. Had a nice breakfast, later my eyes were closed, listening to Frank Sinatra on the iPod, when the Doc shook my toe at around 9am.

My labs showed my blood was back to minimum norms, infection was down, and unbelievably I was able to kick the problem overnight, when it normally takes days. What a blessing.

So I went home. Had two days of feeling like I had been beaten up, Sunday feeling reasonably good again, and back in the saddle on Monday.

Cancer is tricky. I have a blood draw the day before every chemo treatment. That means my blood was good a week ago, I had a chemo treatment the next day, and within 5 days was in trouble. Of course I was four rounds of chemo into the cycle, and it is also cumulative - which has an impact.

I feel lucky there were no other complications, and I got though this relatively easy.

Tomorrow morning I have a PET scan scheduled, which will reveal what mean Mr. Cancer is up to.

Wednesday I get the official results, but will read the radiology myself on Tuesday to get a sense of what is happening. Of course my hopes are that I am in remission again, and can put round four of cancer in the history books. I hope for that because I don't like the alternative.

I will let you know. In the meantime I am doing fine.

God's Blessings.

Wednesday, February 27, 2013 - Round Four in the History Books

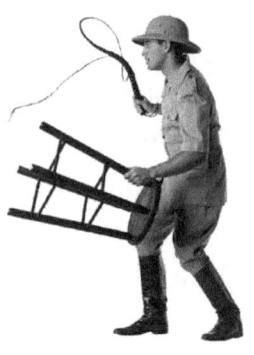

I just spent about 2 hours with Sam. The great news is the results from the PET scan and the radiologist that read them, is that I am not only in remission, but have made significant progress. Tumors are inactive, significantly smaller, or gone.

My blood counts have climbed back up and are in the green. I am getting better!

But, it is clear that if I follow the same path I have been on for the last 2.5 years, I will be fighting round five of cancer by summer, I will be ill from chemo, and the whole cycle will just repeat. If I never try something different, this cycle will just continue until eventually my body will ignore the chemo, and some very unpleasant things begin to happen that will kill me.

So it is time to get out of the box. While cancer is so inert at the moment, we are going to start radiation. I will go through it 5 weeks, 5 days a week. The prize is that at the conclusion of that, it is not unreasonable to believe that I could be in remission for a year or two.

Now is the time for me to buck up, and get through this next phase. If it works the way we believe it will, I will have an extended break from the chaos of cancer. I would be very grateful for that.

While I am not looking forward to radiation, the potential benefits are very exciting.

Oh yeah, I also have to see a cardiologist because of the blood pressure issues I am having, which likely is just the chemo, but we want to be sure.

I will update everyone on news as I get it.

God's Blessings to all of you.

Thursday, March 7, 2013 - Grateful and Growing

Just like anyone with cancer, my mission in life has changed from all of the things I was doing before cancer, to helping others with cancer, just get through as easily as possible. Especially in the beginning of cancer there is lots of fear and uncertainty. It' really scared me! I would like to minimize that for others as much as possible.

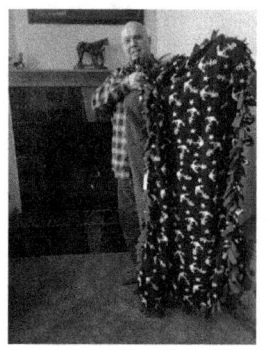

To accomplish that, I have been writing for the last two and a half years. I write a blog on my own web site, I wrote a book, Prospering with Cancer, and I have really tried to get, in marketing terms, reach.

When I first started writing my blog, when all of my family and friends thought I was facing immanent death, I was getting hundreds of hits on each blog published. Over the last 2.5 years that has dropped off to a trickle. Not that people don't care, it just becomes an old and maybe boring story for them.

That made me realize I was catering to the wrong audience for my goal. That's when I found the Blog for a Cure website. There, I witnessed how much people with cancer care and want to support others. The support we all receive on this site is inspirational at a minimum. I am grateful, as we all are, for that.

In that I have run global marketing campaigns for many years, I guess somewhere in my genes I just wanted to kick it up another notch, and hopefully get an even broader reach.

On a personal note, I have just gone into remission for the fourth time. With that in mind the Docs have decided it would be good to double down.

To that end, I will begin Radiation next week for the first time. It will be every weekday for six weeks. I will also be taking xeloda, an oral form or 5FU. They think it is not unreasonable to think that I can stay in remission for a year after doing this. So that would be a very exciting blessing too, if that is the way it works out.

God's Blessings to all of you.

Saturday, March 23, 2013 - 4 Bullets Fired, Still Alive and Doing Well

"If we are facing in the right direction, all we have to do is keep on walking." **- Buddhist Proverb**

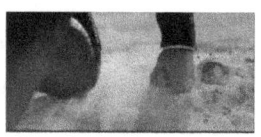

Any bout with cancer is tough, getting through 4 rounds is an accomplishment. For me, I think the mental challenge is larger than the physical challenge, and the physical challenge isn't easy, which is the point. With the constant issue of what is physically lost in health, stamina, and ability to do ordinary things, there is a real mental shift I believe must happen to be able to happily deal with the new reality. I can't overstate this; it is without a doubt the key most important attribute to maintaining a strong positive mental position. One has to let go of the past, and find ways to obtain joy for the new reality. The faster a person can accept their current reality, the better.

Of course everyone and their personal experiences will vary. My situation is one reality; I have seen and met people who are far worse, as well as much better. No matter where one is with their personal challenges, finding a positive path is essential to maximizing the best potential outcome. Negative energy and sour attitudes that lead to stress, have no healing properties, and in fact studies have shown healing is impaired.

That is the point of the Buddhist Proverb, but I would add that the faster you can find the right path and then follow it the better. So how do you do that?

From a personal point of view I recommend you have a strong faith in God to be leading you, and taking care of you, so you can be relieved of the worry of life in general. The next important step is to find a medical team you click with and that you can trust. If either are not working, fire them and find one you can trust.

If you are freshly diagnosed with cancer you are likely frightened and don't know what to do.

That's where SU2C can really help. They know the ropes, and they are connected to every organization that counts. Minimally, they have people that can give you advice and direction, which will greatly improve the speed of you getting onto the right track. When it comes to cancer, you don't have time to fool around. Your life, and the quality of it, is dependent on fast and effective action. Maybe you are the type that wants to control everything, and that translates to you doing it on your own. So be it. Few amateurs go to Vegas and come back rich. Personally I would recommend you find the resources that have the most efficient and rapid path to resolution, and that means getting some experienced guidance.

Realize also that all cancer treatment regimes are shared via the web among all related medical professions. While well intending people will tell you have to go to a prestigious institution to get effective treatment, I will politely disagree. So long as your doctors are paying attention to all of the latest and greatest treatments, learning, and following best practices, the treatment you can receive locally can be equal to any of the best.

Case in point, I have beaten the statistical odds, and am doing relatively well. I have beaten four rounds of metastatic colorectal cancer. Even though I am technically in remission, my medical team knows if we just wait, I will be in my fifth round of cancer this summer. So instead of waiting for that, I am now taking chemo (5FU) and radiation. They think there is a real chance of me being in remission for much longer than just a few months now. We shall see. The point is – they are thinking and are out of the box. The bigger point is that I am still alive because of them and they are a local team in a small town in Colorado. No matter, they are a really great team, and I am grateful beyond words.

Please, if you, or someone you know is new to cancer, get on it fast. Don't jump around looking for something better. If you get plugged into the right resources in the beginning, there isn't anything better, so find a team you trust.

Your time should be spent following the plan, making everyday count, and appreciating the things that matter.

Sunday, March 31, 2013 - Time to Live

"And in the end, it's not the years in your life that count. It's the life in your years."
- Abraham Lincoln

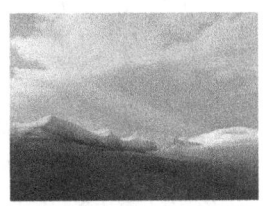

What does it mean to live? When is the right time to live? When are you doing the things that count? Is life meant to be "willy-nilly flowing," or are we born to accomplish larger and more specific goals? If so, then what are they? What gives you a sense of accomplishment? Have you noticed what you measure as important changes with time?

Is anybody born aware of these questions? I doubt it. But one of the inevitable developments of life is to eventually understand that life is simultaneously precious and precarious, and the things one does in this life matter. I believe free will is vital for good people to thrive. All people are free to choose as they will, which results in people that will contribute, others that will take, and some that will only damage.

However people also change. Some through the slow but inescapable shaping of a soul in lessons both good and bad, others because of some momentous event. Whichever the path, the outcome can be either profoundly joyous or sad. If only this epiphany were known in the beginning of life's journey, it could either serve to validate the course you are on, or awaken you to the need to change. But the reality is that it is the journey that sets the limits on values we learn, and ultimately the people we become.

One of life's true pities is that some are so absorbed they will never achieve an awakening leading to a higher sense of value for human or even spiritual compassion and value. On the other hand, for whatever causes an awakening, when the moment finally comes, it is a blessing to realize what really matters and what you really need to do, before time runs out.

I wish everyone could experience that moment in time, to know the importance of how personal priorities impact what kind of a person you will ultimately be. If that is not seen as pleasing, I also wish you would have enough time to make things right for yourself and the people you care about.

The blessing of a life threatening illness like cancer, is in potentially having the time to think through all of this. In a sudden death, time just runs out, and you are left wherever you are in life's journey. Life's objectives are either complete, satisfying, and settled, or they are not – final curtain.

For many on the cancer journey, it will serve to become the momentous event that causes deep self-reflection, which will inspire us to settle all of what the book of life has written as unsettled events, at least to that point. We will strive to resolve and prepare a final chapter that ultimately closes with what we see as a happy and positive ending, at least to the extent that is possible.

The motivation to do good works and help others is not limited to just cancer patients; it also inspires many of our family and friends. The world is a running river full of people that have equally realized though association of those afflicted by cancer, that life matters. They become strongly committed to minimize suffering, improve the quality of life, and provide joy for everyone, through acts of good will, unbridled generosity, and gracious kindness.

They reflect the very best of humanity. These works are from generous hearts and souls motivated to serve and improve the life of others less fortunate. Often, it is their gift of love that gives others comfort, time to live, time to find joy, time to resolve, time to settle everything, and time to shape their final chapter to spiritually full and rich conclusions.

While many are talking about end of life conversations, a topic that needs serious attention to be sure, it also makes sense to sort out what happens before that conversation, when mortality is evident and you still have a chance to make a difference.

It is immeasurably humbling to be the object of such rich human generosity from people I have known all my life to literally strangers.

God will richly bless all that give, so others can live.

Monday, April 8, 2013 - Cancer's Path to God's Light

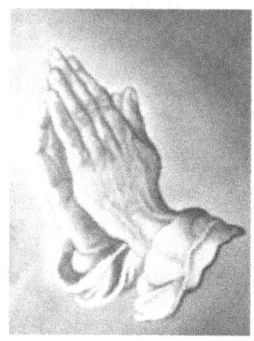

All of us are close to cancer. We all know someone, or have had the experience ourselves. I have been in the battle for 2 years, 7 months, 12 days and as you know have been open and have communicated the journey. That has acted like a bit of light, as I have had numerous conversations with cancer patients, friends have also asked me to talk to new cancer patients they know.

One of those conversations began 5 months and 9 days ago with a young lady that had just learned she had bladder cancer. Today I learned that her cancer has metastasized to her liver and lymph nodes. She has been told she has months to live.

Nobody knows how deep the well of courage and love is inside of us, until we tap into it. It seems that it ordinarily only happens when a momentous event like facing cancer and the likelihood of death occur. When that happens, you will see and feel the courage, and the love God inspires within humanity.

She posted the news on Facebook to let everyone know the news today. She opened her thoughts with inspirational words of thanks for the love and support she has received as well as some advise, in essence sharing the idea of loving thy neighbor. Her thoughts are so beautiful, courageous and loving.

That inspiration well exists in all but a very few. You tap into it when you are sharing your love and support with the people that are afflicted with this retched thieving disease. But I think that God knows that the well is even deeper, in fact much deeper. When we are tasked with undertaking the rigors of a life depriving disease, knowing that death is perhaps near, most will find it to be a catalyst to reflect back on all of your years to sort out what really matters. Age and experience is a natural basses for this maturing in learning, but nothing will speed it along like the news that you have cancer.

Once people get over the shock of knowing that they must deal with the disease, and have sorted out doctors, treatment and so on, there is time to think. That seems to accelerate the understanding of God's plan like nothing else. People glow with peace and love. I wish all of humanity could get a dose of where this accelerated perspective takes us that have glimpsed or experienced it's depths. If all of humanity were able to achieve God's loving position as demonstrated by my friend, the world would be that much closer to heaven.

In the meanwhile, we can appreciate the depth of the courageous loving souls that demonstrate the compassion and beauty we are all capable of. God leads us all toward that loving light at the speed that is right.

I wish God's blessing to my friend Kimberley and her family. You have fought bravely, and shared love wisely. May we all follow your leadership. Thanks for the inspiration you share.

Tuesday, April 16, 2013 - My Last BLOG

"If you are brave enough to say goodbye, life will reward you with a new hello." - *Unknown*

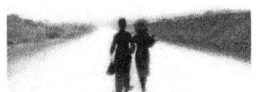

No, I am not dying – at least not yet.

When I discovered I had cancer, I prayed a lot. I felt there was a calling for me to take some of the communication skills I have learned along the way, and try to use them to help others. To that end, I very transparently wrote about the experience as a way to try to help others find a positive outlook, alleviate fear, and set a context that would not only help them as an individual, but also all of their circle of family, friends, and colleagues.

It seems that there have been some successes in doing that.

At the same time and from the beginning, I felt that if this communication was in fact a divine calling, that things would sort of take off, and I would be busy with the message in various ways. I also felt that if this was just me thinking I should do these things, that not much would come of it. Well, from my point of view - not much has come of it, so I guess it was just me trying to do something good.

There are lots of people that have cancer and many of them have written books, or have gotten involved in various activities to help others along the way. All of these things are good, valuable, and noble.

I just don't have the feeling that I have really made much difference, and truly, don't think much more will come from it.

I think it is time to let the people that do seem to have a voice in all of this carry the torch.

As such, I am retiring my philosophical and personal perspective on the rigors of cancer. I plan to discontinue posting blogs. If God has other plans for me, I'm sure he will let me know.

To all that have followed, thank you, and God's blessings to all.

Friday, April 19, 2013 - Mistakes are the Portals of Discovery

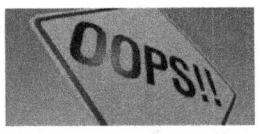

The vacuum of silence is a great place for imagination to run amuck. It also illustrates the point that a cancer patient, intentionally or not can develop feelings of isolation. It seems impossible for that to happen as I am constantly in contact with family, friends, colleagues, and medical teams, yet it did.

I have just learned something about me and about you. First about me. You have undoubtedly noticed that my writing has shifted away from how I am getting along with cancer as a primary focus. One of the main motivations behind that is that I really dislike listening to the endless droning of a person's issues with their lack of health. It just bores me to death. That is probably a failing inside me as a compassionate human. It's not that I don't care about people, nor does it indicate a lack of concern. But the minute details of health gripes are more than what I can stay engaged in for very long.

Yet, I have also noticed that I have become far more compassionate when I am with other cancer patients. I suspect it is because I better understand the issues they care about, and feel empathetic and a sense of wanting to help them.

Insofar as my own gripes, I decided a long time ago, that I would avoid too much detail about what is going on with me, because I assumed your interest in my issues would soon get boring. I actually think there is only a certain amount you can stand still. But I made a basic marketing mistake. As views on my website dropped off, I realized that I was writing to the wrong audience, which is why I started writing for "Blog for a Cure." The problem that I didn't see was that I was now addressing an audience that is really eager to know about the cancer experience as well as the inspirational messages.

So after some coaching and enlightenment from my friends, I am going to add cancer experience thinking to the blogs.

As such, here is a quick review of my last 4.5 months.

I have gone through a full course of Full Fury chemo to get into remission in round 4 of metastatic colorectal cancer, which is also in my lungs. I got to experience (once again) a host of chemo related issues:

- Migraine headaches strong enough that only the combination of morphine and large doses of ibuprofen could make tolerable

- Constant nausea, and fatigue that you can't communicate effectively

- Feeling that your whole body is ill, also something that you can't communicate effectively

- A trip to emergency via ambulance for a neutropenic fever with shaking that looked like Parkinson's disease, because my white blood cell count cratered. Spent the night in the hospital

- I won't describe the GI issues because you don't want to know

- But I can tell you it involves bleeding and pain that is brutal

When I finished chemo and went into remission, I went straight into radiation, and continued one variety of chemo - Fluorouracil or 5-FU.

The first week was tolerable. By the second week I was getting very ill and pain was increasing. By the fourth week I was far too ill to be able to tolerate radiation and chemo, so I discontinued the chemo and continued with radiation. Pain levels are brutal, I refused morphine because I wanted to maintain my ability to think. By the 21st treatment out of 30, the pain levels reached a point that almost had me blacking out, I couldn't make it to the morphine fast enough. I have been taking morphine daily now for four days. I intend to continue for at least another week. I have four more radiation treatments remaining, and will finish Thursday of next week (April 25th).

I have become short tempered, and have at times emotionally struggled with how I am going to get through this. It is a very mental game to continue, knowing the consequences of treatment, yet it's impossible to stop, knowing that it could provide enough time for someone to actually find a cure for what will otherwise kill me. This is the largest conundrum of my life. I think you can see why I have not focused on this in my writing. It just feels like my problem, not yours.

Finally, about you. I have learned that some of you have benefited from the philosophical perspective I have journeyed though, as a way of helping you understand issues you or someone you know face. I am so grateful that it has created that benefit. Others have benefited from helping them understand the road ahead, as their largest challenge in the beginning of the cancer journey - is fear of the unknown. Many people have expressed their desire for me to continue, and so I will.

I have always written with the ultimate desire to find a way to help people, friends have deepened this understanding, and coach me to also write about the challenges of the disease as well, which I am going to do. Cancer patients and professionals like SU2C thrive among the finest human spirit the planet offers. They represent a talented group of people that not only care for those with cancer, they have also taken action to bestow great works and contributions to people that really need help. It seems to be the perfect example of "love thy neighbor." I am lucky to be in the company of giants.

I would add this, if you ponder any aspect of cancer you don't understand, or would just like to read some thinking on a particular topic, then please let me know. I would be thrilled to address the challenges that you face to the extent that I can. I always want to share. I want to help, and I especially want to repay the kind support I have received though my attempt to pay it forward.

God bless the caregivers and interested souls that contribute so much, and God's blessings and health to those that battle the disease.

Sunday, April 21, 2013 - "When we put a limit on what we will do, we put a limit on what we can do."

– Charles Schwab

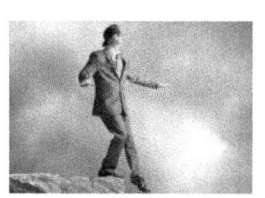

I was not prepared for the rigors of radiation. It deceived me a bit. Of course none of the medical types really know what your experience is going to be. They neither want to under nor over sell you, which makes sense; they really can't predict how your experience will be.

They gave me some vague ideas, along with a document I had to sign that had a long list of things that can go wrong, which alone should be enough to want to skip the whole thing. But you know how lawyer speak is. When I listen to the myriad drugs that are advertised on television, with all of the caveats, who would want to take any of them? So I had a bit of hesitation but no big concerns. I also read accounts on both sides of the fence. For some it was a "cake-walk," for others a problem.

Here is what I experienced. First, my medical team thought they were doing their very best by having me take radiation and chemo at the same time. Chemo is great at creating pain and causing suffering all by itself. They knew that radiation created many of the same symptoms, but because the chemo component for this plan was a small part of what I normally took, just 5-FU, they thought I would tolerate it well, and it would also enhance the radiation. Insofar as my tolerance for this - no way! I didn't have a chance to get over the previous round

*of six full-fury chemo treatments. So I started off
sick from chemo and it just got worse from there.
Except for one new element – PAIN, in big doses.*

*But I can't back out. The big prize is that radiation is
often used as a curative treatment, and in
particular, it could cure the rectal cancer and stop
the on and off cycles I have been going through for
2.7 years. While it is still in my lungs, it doesn't seem
to be doing much. That's what changed the doctors'
mind and lead them to start radiation. They
initially thought the lung cancer would kill me
before the rectal cancer became a problem, so they
treated me with chemo to attack all the cancer that
was freely running around my body as well as the
specific sites. But lung cancer didn't kill me and it
hasn't shown up any place else, so they decided to do
something more aggressive about the rectal cancer.*

*Radiation therapy uses high-energy radiation to kill
cancer cells by damaging it's DNA. It will also kill
normal cells. For me, it is causing enough damage
to cause bleeding, and a brutally painful sensitive
tumor site. The idea is as your body repairs what is
damaged, normal cells grow back.*

*This treatment has created two difficult mental
challenges, the first is just mustering the motivation
to go in and take the radiation, and the other is
going to the bathroom and suffering the pain. Both
have to be done, mentally I want to retract and do
neither. It is difficult to go do what you dread.*

*However, my big hope is that I can hang around
long enough to have a cure show up. There are some
remarkable things that have been happening.*

While chemo and radiation are treatments that shut-off a person's immune systems, for years, researchers have been trying to figure out a way to kill cancer cells by using a patient's immune system. In August of 2011 the University of Pennsylvania School of Medicine claimed a victory in that effort.

Doctors removed a billion T-cells from a 65-year-old man - a type of white blood cell that fights viruses and tumors, and gave them new genes that would program the cells to attack his cancer, which was leukemia. The altered cells were infused back into his veins.

At first, nothing happened. But after 10 days, all hell broke loose in his hospital room. He began shaking with chills and his temperature shot up. His blood pressure fell like a rock. He was so ill that doctors moved him into intensive care and warned that he might die. His family gathered at the hospital, fearing the worst. A few weeks later, the fevers were gone, and so was the leukemia. There was no trace of it anywhere.

They said that this form of treatment is like giving a scent to a bloodhound. The T-cells had been given the scent of the leukemia cells and they go out and hunt them down. The hope is to give T-cells the scent of colon cancer, breast cancer, lung cancer and train them go out and kill all kinds of cancers. While it is dangerous, and only being done in Universities, it is nevertheless a breakthrough. By the way, they have tried it on colorectal cancer patients as well, one of them died. This treatment can create what is known as a cytokine storm.

Whenever a disease is present in a body, part of the response of a body to mount a defense, is triggered by effected cells that secrete a substance called a "Cytokine". Cytokines are small cell-signaling protein molecules that are secreted by numerous cells and are a category of signaling molecules used extensively in intercellular communication. The term "cytokine" has been used to refer to the immunomodulating agents, such as interleukins and interferons. Cytokines enhance cellular immune responses, which favor antibody responses.

Cytokine storms were the main cause of death in the 1918 "Spanish Flu" pandemic. Cytokine storm deaths are weighted more heavily towards people with healthy immune systems, due to its ability to produce stronger immune responses, like increasing cytokine levels.

For now I am trapped. I have four more to go, I give serious thought to not doing them, yet I have to. This is the most difficult mental challenge of my life. I have to do something I really don't want to do. I don't know how I will get it done; I just know that I will – because I have to. If I don't do this, the amount of living I have left will be cut short. I doubt that there are many decisions that are more difficult, with larger consequences.

Welcome to cancer, where decisions aren't easy, and stakes are huge. Just remember, you can do it alone, or you can enlist the people that are there to help you.

May God guide your decisions.

Sunday, May 5, 2013 - Hitting a Brick Wall on Purpose Hurts

Dealing with the mechanics of cancer is a challenge all by itself. Lot's of visits to the doctor/hospital and lots of treatments, blood draws etc. All of these things are physical and tangible. In some ways they are even easy to manage. You can more or less see them, touch them, and manage them.

What's not so obvious is the emotional and physiological turmoil treading just below the surface. A fairly broad range of disturbance is constantly tugging at your otherwise normal thinking and feelings. Fear, anger, uncertainty, doubts, and anxiety all demand attention. All of that while you are weak, ill, and possibly in minor to horrifying levels of pain.

These factors are just too persuasive and present to ignore. They can reshape your personality for periods of time. Woe be onto those that are nearby, such as a caregiver, because this monster can lead you to suspend manners and respect which can make you unpleasant to be around.

Who would choose that? How much of your life have you spent in giving consideration to working well with the social settings you are exposed to? Probably more than you realize. We are always working on that. We are always looking for ways to be more socially effective. Yet the cancer monster seems to be able to suspend all of that at times, as the level of internal strife becomes louder than everything that is going on around you. Sometimes the mental noise level of suffering just drains our attention, lowering tolerance for everything to levels so low that what you might ordinarily barely notice, now becomes something that just makes your anger flash.

It defies everything we know about living life constrained in ways that allow a pleasant experience for everybody. Cancer can suddenly transport us back to the social skills of a two year old, barely able to tolerate the easiest of social challenges. We know better, we don't really desire to be lunatics, but this monster can bring it out.

With all of that said, at times I have been left with shame and or embarrassment for being a jerk. I don't really believe saying, "sorry I have cancer and I'm in pain," is a "get out of jail" excuse. All my life I have taught myself to take responsibility for my actions. I don't want to abuse any relationship. But the reality is that there have been times when my ability to maintain the rigor of social intelligence has completely failed me and I have barked when I should have bitten my lip or just been quite.

The challenge of cancer is more than just getting to the doctor, there can be significant emotional and physiological challenges as well. I think those issues are more difficult to seek help for. I haven't. I keep thinking I can take care of everything. I am at the backend of some incredibly difficult times, I am beaten up physically, dealing with lots of pain, and believe my emotional intellect has also been damaged, or at least suffered from temporary stupidity at times.

People that get through these things, seem to have inspirational thoughts to share about what they have gained overall. A deep understanding of the values of life emerge, along with an enthusiasm to share the insights, and help others along the way.

But, it is difficult to understand your strength as a cancer warrior when you are bloodied from battle. Of course you know how much you have gone through, what you may not know is how much is left, and if you have what it takes to get through that. I can tell you I hit a brick wall a few weeks ago, and for the first time in my life, could not see how I was going to get to the end, in this case, of the radiation treatments. I couldn't escape the pain, and I didn't feel like I could quit, unless I was willing to accept an accelerated death. Not an easy mental position. I'm not a good example of what you should do, because I did nothing. I just kept going, but suffered rough physiological edges. No doubt the councilors that were offered could have helped me cope with the situation, but I was to tuff for that. In hindsight, I was foolish. I would recommend that if you find yourself hitting the brick wall, you accept the help.

Really, if you are standing there wondering if you can make it through, you may want to let the people that train to help others help you.

They just might be able to make getting through easier.

Wednesday, May 22, 2013 - The Latest and Greatest

I saw both of my oncology doctors today. They believe I am over the hump, and should make major progress in recovery over the next two weeks. I have another PET scan scheduled for July 3rd to make sure everything is clear, for the time being. However, both doctors believe I may well be out of the woods for years now!

Of course there are never guarantees with cancer, but this is the best news I have received since the whole episode started nearly 3 years ago!

Hoorah!! I think the ice cream helped.

Dairy Queen anyone?

Perhaps my eternal optimism is unbalanced.

I am reminded that I still have cancer in my lungs that is active, it could go other places, there are no guarantees, mileage will vary, etc. It is possible that cancer will migrate to my brain, liver or wherever. I am still technically stage IV terminal.

However, I choose to look at the good news, and not worry about the rest. Staying positive throughout this has served me well, and I will continue to do that!

Sunday, June 2, 2013 - The Road Ahead

"It is literally true that you can succeed best and quickest by helping others to succeed."

- Napoleon Hill

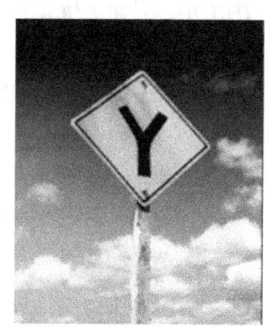

My battle with terminal metastatic colorectal cancer has lasted nearly three years. Because cancer metastasized to my lungs, in the beginning I was told to not expect more than a year and a half of remaining life. It was a difficult wake up call, which motivated deep and accelerated introspective evaluation. It rapidly crystalized the differences between the things in life that really matter versus all of the things that simply don't. I concluded the lessons of life that have value in the end, are about people, love, and the grace of God from which all good comes. It is because of these exceedingly simply, yet powerfully profound awakenings, that I am grateful to cancer. I believe it has made me a better person through really hard lessons.

The uncertainty of the journey has been one of the more disturbing experiences. In the beginning it was not knowing how horrible the progression of the disease would be to experience. It was the fear of what would happen to my family. The void of understanding for what would actually kill me, and what that experience would be. How would my family be impacted? Have I made a difference in this life that mattered?

Those uncertainties yielded way to the treatment regime. That led to not knowing what to expect from chemo. I had to discover that it was a down hill slope that gets worse over time. I had no idea how sick I would be. I had no idea how sick I could be.

But I stayed positive, I focused on what gave me joy, I didn't quit, and I never gave up or in, ever. I got through it. Yet, because it is cancer it came back, again, and again, and again. Four times I have battled back the infernal progression of a deadly disease that attacks slowly but surely.

With each attack, my compassion has grown along with my desire to help others get through the journey. This disease is so difficult that everyone that is exposed to it, ultimately just wants to help others. It taps the core of human compassion and drives people to reach out with a personal desire to urgently render any and all aid. The core of what is ugly in cancer, causes the best of humanity to blossom. It's a beautiful and amazing thing to watch.

Round four of cancer is in the history books for me now. The last bout required 111 continuous days of a combination of chemo and radiation, and raised the bar of personal challenge to get through it, to levels that were exceedingly difficult, and unmatched by a country mile to anything I have ever experienced.

Of course I never want to return to that, and the doctors have actually given me a pretty bright prognosis. But it is still cancer, and it looks for ways to return, and it too never gives up trying.

There are armies of people working to unravel the mysteries of this disease. There are astonishing discovers constantly found. There is no doubt that someday the barbaric suffering caused by this disease will be viewed as an ugly historical event. But not today.

So while I am feeling better every day, and working to return to my former self, somewhere ahead of me, there is a fork in the road. Down one direction, cancer kills both of us, down the other - a cure is found, cancer dies, and death has to wait for some other cause. The uncertainty I now live with, is not knowing how far down the road the fork is. I hope it is far enough away for science to reveal the secrets that cancer has hidden throughout time, and we can finally kill this monster.

Until then, the generosity of human spirit will continue to seek ways to cure or comfort all that struggle and suffer.

That is a reflection of the spirit of God, for which I am awed and grateful.

I pray for a cure, and comfort for all.

Sunday, June 30, 2013 - Waiting for News

"Health is the greatest gift, contentment the greatest wealth, faithfulness the best relationship." - Buddha

From January 2nd until April 23 (111 continuous days), I was either on chemo or chemo and radiation. It was a very challenging experience to get through physically and emotionally.

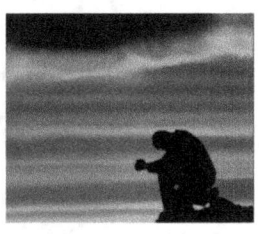

I have been out of treatment now for nine weeks, and have only been feeling reasonable for the last two.

Tuesday (July 3rd) I have another PET (Positron Emission Tomography) scan to find out how I am doing. Hopefully they will find that I am cancer free and I can go on with recovery. If they discover active cancer, I will be back in chemo and or radiation within two weeks.

I am easily able to rationalize why I am OK, but in the end, the reality of the story has nothing to do with how I rationalize it. Cancer has a life of it's own despite my best intentions, desires, and hopes. Cancer at its most basic level blindly seeks to live, to grow and to thieve. It is unaware that it's goals for greatness, are ultimately what will kill it, and the person hosting it.

The battle of cancer is an odd battle with a part of yourself, a dark and evil duality of purpose. We both strive to thrive, one or both of us has to die.

So once again from this three-year battle, I wait for the test and the pronouncement that will soon follow on July 3rd 2013.

I will soon find myself striving to increase my level of health with a feeling that the radiation I suffered through paid off, or I will find myself in the thick of the battle for my life once more.

Tick-tock, which will it be?

Thursday, July 4, 2013 - Reach Deeper, that wasn't Enough

"Adversity causes some men to break; others to break records."
- William Ward

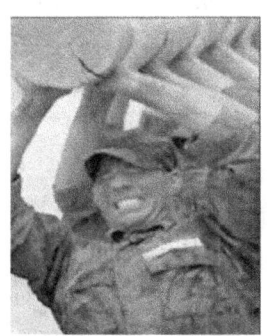

Frankly, I am not happy about the news; cancer is back.

There is some perspective here. The good news is that the rectal cancer is completely gone. Which means the radiation I suffered through was successful. The bad news is that the cancer in my lungs is thriving, growing, and expanding.

That really is bad news. Again, a little balance here, it's not a summer fire that is out of control. So we arrive at the issue, we have to jump on the cancer in my lungs now, rapidly, and aggressively, or I will get to experience an escalating set of bad health related issues.

Colon cancer arrived in my lungs via blood supply. My blood supply can carry it anywhere else in my body, with my liver being a primary concern. Even if it didn't metastasize again, and we just left the cancer in my lungs alone, it could kill me in a relatively short period of time, like six months.

So that's not going to happen.

I am weary of sickness. Emotionally it is just difficult to put the armor back on and head out to war. It's not like I am standing safely in the trenches and operating weapons of war from a safe position. This is more like a hand-to-hand combat. It's up close and personal, and I take a lot of blows. Lose focus, slow down too much, or quit, and you're dead. Now do that every single day for months at a time, and you begin to appreciate the emotional challenge. If your goal is to stay alive, you have to find a way to truly want to win. It has to be a fountain of inspiration that never runs dry, and always keeps you replenished for your ultimate goal – winning.

I have been battle tested in the last almost three years. I have been seriously beaten up, yet I have so far ultimately prevailed in the battle for my life. I thought the war was over for a while, but true to life, the alarm has been raised, and the call to action form my fifth skirmish has unexpectedly arrived once more.

It is easy to feel that I have already given this all I have. It reminds me of American Special Forces. What makes them so amazing is their training of course. The most valuable benefit from their training is being taught that they have a deeper reservoir of fight in them than they ever knew existed. Their training teaches them how to draw on that to overcome what appears to be far more than is possible for them or for humans in general. They discover a deeper richer reserve of fight, tap it, use it, adapt, and overcome.

And so it is for me right now. I have to find a way to reach even deeper to find even more fight, so that I may apply it to the challenges I am now facing.

Starting today I have more battles, more physical, and more emotional challenges to conquer.

I don't want to, I have to.

May God supply all of us with the strength we need to win the battles we must.

Round 5

Saturday, August 3, 2013 - What's in your Glass?

"Courage is not the absence of fear, but rather the judgment that something else is more important than fear." -James Neil Hollingworth

Next week I begin treatment for round 5 of cancer. I can imagine a girl walking around a boxing ring with a sign displaying the number 5 carried above her head.

I am in a prizefight, and so far the battle has been worthy of a championship bout. Each round the combatants have dished out punishment, both are bloodied.

Now the two opponents are sitting in their corners with trainers cooing out encouragement, bravado and courage while wounds are treated and sweat is wiped away. In a ten thousand yard stare, their eyes meet and are locked, absent from blinking, partly to signal no fear in hopes of gaining a psychological edge for the next round. The other to assess their own fears quickly - mentally shoring up weaknesses that can weaken their fight, which could result in a decreasing probability of winning not only the round, but also the battle.

The battle can be won or lost on mental attitude, strength, commitment, and pure unwavering resolve to be the victor. This does not mean that a cancer warrior does not have fear. Only a fool is not afraid. Fear too is an enemy. The measure of courage is not whether you are afraid, it is what you do when you are. It is the difference between cowards and heroes. Courage is the ability to act when gripped with fear. It is the commitment to keep going when you aren't sure of your ability or the outcome. It is caring more about the people around you than you care for yourself.

Sometimes courage is in you but never seen, because circumstances never cause courage to act. Sometimes circumstances call on courage, but it hides behind fear, needing the encouragement of some motivating circumstance or person to help it to spring forth into action.

It seems there is a shorter path to courage for those who always have a glass that is filled, versus those that see the glass partially empty. More than half the battle is the perception of the odds of winning, and not dwelling too deeply on all of the issues that can harm you. For those that are focused on only the fears and dangers, the path to victory is obscured. If you can't see a successful conclusion, it is difficult to manage your way to success.

When the bell rings you can bet there are going to be some punishing blows. Cancer delves out lots of punishment. Crushing punishment. You have to have your battle face on when the bell sounds, because it's going to get rough.

A normal human, doesn't sit ringside to watch people get hurt. People are drawn to the championship fights, for one reason. We all love to see a winner. We love winners that overcome great challenges. We feel the crushing punishment as it plays out in front of us. We measure how we as individuals would react. We feel the pain, fear, fatigue, and how desperate the situation is. Round after round after round of watching terrorizing punishment, we are thrilled to ecstatic elation when the person we are rooting for pulls out a victory. Multiple that when that person is someone you love.

When that person fights the good fight and loses regardless, we are proud of their commitment to have the courage and commitment to stay in a battle that as individuals we are not sure we could endure. That makes us proud of them as well, and often martyrizes our feeling for them.

Not every person is able to rise above the suffering and fear in cancer to fight with noble character. In reality I feel most sorry for them. For they miss the deeper lessons of understanding in just how generous and noble humanity is. They miss the humble lessons of God's love. They ultimately miss the beauty and precious offering of abundant love, care, and beauty of things around them.

May God give all the warriors the vision to see beyond the personal battles, and the strength to find courage to win the battles they must.

Saturday, August 24, 2013 - Three years, and still Grateful

I am grateful for . .

Today is the three-year anniversary of an event that changed the course of my life. While on a business trip to California, I learned I have cancer.

It has become increasingly apparent there are ways to look at this that are just loaded with miserable thinking, and there are ways to look at it from a perspective that has allowed me to prosper and grow as an individual and in faith.

The key difference seems to be how one chooses to witness an event. I have a long list of things that I have lost. Things that were important to me, and things that I thought of as a part of the very definition of who I am, or wanted to be. I have lost many abilities, which too, massively changed the sort of things I can and want to do, versus the things I am now realistically only able to do.

But through it all, I nevertheless have come to realize that what I am left with is the most valuable of all. I have faith in God's work and plan, I have a much greater appreciation for what life offers, I have my family, and I have friends. For those things I am grateful beyond words.

One would never expect cancer to be the perfect conclusion to your senior years. But if it is cancer that was required for helping me achieve a perspective that is aligned with the vision that God seeks for all of humanity to have, love thy neighbor and believe in me, than this is the perfect event in my life. The value of this lesson is greater than any other I have experienced. I am grateful to be here, I am grateful for the lesson and I am grateful for the loving support I have received from more people than I feel I deserve.

May the love of God guide your life richly.

Saturday, September 7, 2013 - Far from Stranded

"The optimist lives on the peninsula of infinite possibilities; the pessimist is stranded on the island of perpetual indecision."
- William Arthur Ward

The difference between victory and defeat sometimes is nothing more than how you perceive it. Am I stranded with a terminal disease, or am I free to explore regions of life I would have otherwise never seen?

I never have liked the feeling of hopelessness. Ever. I have always looked for a way to find the roses when walking in beds of thorns. It's a perspective, and it has greatly added to the richness of my life. Just like all of us, there have been times that I have found myself in situations that were just not happy. Yet, there has always been an option for somehow changing the situation to resolve discontent. Sometimes it was an external influence that had to be modified, and sometimes the trouble was inside of me. It isn't always easy to recognize the problem when it is internal. I think the normal person tends to look for trouble on the inside last. I have observed some people that have from appearances, never looked inside; they are the people that seem to be least content with the world around them.

I find the situation I am in now to be very different than any I have previously encountered. This time the problem certainly isn't external; it is definitely an internal issue. Except it isn't a problem created by poor perception, I just happen to have terminal cancer. The model of my life is to change the situation until it is pleasing again. The problem is, I can't get rid of the cancer.

But I am responsible for and capable of changing my perception of what is pleasing. I have had to let go of so much. Stuff I am just unable to do. Many of the things that once were the cornerstone of things to do that were fun, are simply gone.

Yet, I have found a way to more deeply appreciate the spirit of humanity and grow my faith in God. Both of which now seem to be more important than any of the things that I have left behind.

So what is being stranded? A sure path to wilting and dying, or is it a rarefied opportunity to discover some of the secrets of life that have the greatest value one can measure. At the very least it is perception, and a willingness to look inside, and travel through the barriers that would otherwise ensnare you inside of a locked world, which has no hope or joy.

The best parts of humanity have always grown from freedom, hope, love, and joy.

Cancer can take my life it can't reach my spirit. My spirit has done nothing but grow larger, stronger, and more joyful.

The perception from my island is a vast sea of love and joy. Warm breezes, azure sky, white sand, and plenty of time to enjoy the wonder of the view, the company of family and friends, and the love of God.

Won't you join me?

Monday, October 28, 2013 - The Path Unknown

"Once you choose hope, anything's possible." - *Christopher Reeve*

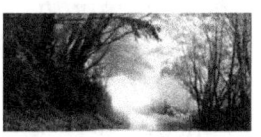

Walking down the path, the difference between fear and adventure is mostly a state of mind. If your life experiences and perceptions have rewarded you with positive outcomes, the path is inviting. Distant turns that are beyond view, are exciting, hold anticipated pleasures, adventures, and discoveries. Memories reward you with lasting pleasure, hopefully shared with someone near you.

I am a creature of habit, and have somehow learned that positive expectations yield positive results. I look for the positive outcomes in everything. I inherently want every experience to have a favorable and memorable outcome. It just leaves me in a happier state of mind, which I prefer.

The question is what happens when the path becomes unknown, uncertain, and probably fatal. Does that or should that really change the way you operate? The way you perceive things? The way you more or less process the experience of things? What you get out of life's offerings?

Oddly, the people I have come to know in the cancer community, seem to largely not only keep their rose colored lens on, they also seem to sharpen. In a way it strikes me as a very odd dichotomy. It's as if life splits into two paths to follow at the same time. The old familiar path that has life's twists, turns and delights is still there and available for exploration and joy. But now the journey also has a new path, the cancer path. My perception is that some days I'm on one, some days the other, and more often than not, it feels like I am on both of them at the same time.

The cancer path can be very un-enjoyable. It can be scary. You can count on being very sick. Yet, because of the amazing people that are there from medical teams, care givers, and other survivors it can also be heart inspiring and warming too. The bifurcated mental oddity has one foot on the cancer path, and the other on Life's path one-step after another. I choose to relate mostly from the path of joy even in the context of living out cancer.

With that in mind, and in that context, here is the status on where the battle is.

I just finished 6 rounds of chemo in the fifth round of cancer. Tuesday the 29th of October (2013) I have a CT scan at 2:15. That will give us the status of how mean Mr. Cancer is doing. I will then meet with my trusty oncologist on Friday to here the rendering. I really don't know what to expect as the next step. It might be; take a rest, it might be; more chemo, it might be; back to radiation.

The cancer path is murky and uncertain. The ultimate outcome is still hanging in the balance between; it kills me, or I actually win and survive. "Survive" meaning cancer goes away and my final cause of death is from something other than cancer. No way to know at this point.

So how does that affect life's journey and the path I am on? At this point – not much. Some days I have no choice but to walk down the uncertainty of cancer's path. Most days I remain on Life's path. Everyday I appreciate Life's abundant gifts and treasures. I think of them, know how precious they are, and remain humbly grateful for the abundance of things I have to still be grateful for.

Life threatening disease is never the likely path we would choose. But if you can find the joyful and valued lessons by habit from the experiences God offers, no matter how scary the path may appear, the are positive outcomes waiting to be discovered and enjoyed.

May God guide you through the everyday joy that is abundantly rich and rewarding.

Thursday, October 31, 2013 - Fighting Beyond Hope

"The only way of discovering the limits of the possible is to venture a little way past them into the impossible." — *Arthur C. Clarke*

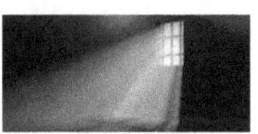

The reality is that more often than not cancer delivers bad news, and so it was today.

For three years I have believed that the spots in my lungs were scare tissue from a spore I caught while in Australia. Today it was confirmed that some 45 lesions are in fact cancer, and have just been too small for the PET scanner to see them. However, the CT scan did.

That means the strategy I have been operating under is no longer valid. I thought that less than a dozen lesions would be attackable by radiation, as I have done in the past. Now — not so.

The reality now is that statistically I have some two years to live. If that turns out to be true for me, then what will kill me is that I get tired of the constant chemo I have to look forward to and stop taking it because I am unhappy with the quality of life, or the chemo stops working and cancer just takes a natural course.

Beyond two years is a function of how stubborn I am, or that a new remedy is discovered that can kill cancer and save my life. Every cancer patient is always hoping for that. Those options are happening with greater frequency, and really, you never know when one will show up. So that is a possibility, who knows what the statistical probability is however.

For me, I am disappointed in today's news. I always thought I had a shot at this, which was within reach. But this news knocks the winning probabilities down to near zero. Maybe it's a bit like loosing the championship game. I have had my heart and soul into winning. Having the game pulled out from underneath me isn't easy.

Yet, my faith in God has never changed. Whatever the path is to get there, I haven't lost a sense of anticipation for what is waiting. Like most people, I just don't like the feeling of a departure. I haven't lost the sense of responsibility for taking care of my family. But, I have also already done all I can do.

I have always said that the battleground for cancer is more mental than it is physical. The advance of this battle has now shifted, and I am challenged to make peace and find comfort with what remains. There is no doubt that will happen, and I must find a way to make that transition rapidly.

From this point forward the fight is about quality, not quantity of life.

My hope is for finding all that offers joy and value in normal day-to-day living. The greatest gift most of us have, is in knowing that it is the love we all share, that is more valuable than even our health. Oddly, it seems that our health challenges only serve to accelerate this understanding.

Today's news is a large accelerant of this lesson for me.

Today, and every day forward, I have to pick myself up and find new inspiration, hope and joy.

God's Blessings to all of you.

Saturday, November 2, 2013 - Making Lemonade

"A man's character is his fate."

- Heraclitus

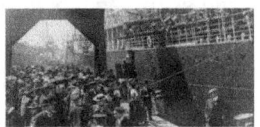

I have had some insights over the last few days and I wanted to share them.

I have come to realize that dying is really as ordinary as ordinary can be. Imagine you could see the world from God's eye. God knows all, sees all. So every person that has ever lived and died is known by God and loved by God.

God watches the miracle of every birth, and the developments of everyone throughout all phases of life – good and bad. Some people are simply jerked from the living by some catastrophic event. Others have time to think about their demise. It is estimated that since 50,000 BC until today, approximately 108 billion people have lived and died on this planet. Let's just say that 90 billion people had the chance to have time to think about their death. God is in your thoughts, and in everyone's thoughts. That means that God has listened to how the thinking of some 90 billion people - went through the thinking development of their death.

Listening to thoughts on what is important, or not. Planning, or not. Sadness, or not. Anger, or not. You get the idea. For certain, patterns have emerged.

It would be really amazing at this point for God to see some fresh new thinking coming out of any human faced with their death. Because of that, it must look fairly unremarkable and ordinary. As ordinary as watching a flower grow have a life of beauty, and eventually wilt away. Its just life. It's expected. It's natural, and it's just what happens.

So here's the interesting dichotomy. There is perhaps a very dispassionate perspective of birth, living and dying, which I have come to believe is the case. To be clear, I believe God loves all of us. God loves the flowers too. But they must all complete the circle of life. It's just the plan and the nature of things.

But, my life matters to me, and it matters to some people in my circle of family and friends. So what is it that is troubling about dying?

It struck me two days ago, and developed a bit more yesterday. It reminded me of the immigrants from Europe destined for America. They left for hope, they sought better opportunities and freedoms. They knew they had a chance for a better future. They anticipated the glory of many new and exciting opportunities to be found in the Promised Land. But there was a moment, when they were on the ship that was being pushed away from the dock. The moment they looked far at the land they were leaving, and they looked close at the people on the dock they would not see again, and they were very sad and very happy at the same time.

The issue I face, and I believe that many have faced, is similar and ordinary from the beginning of time.

I have a strong faith, comfort, and anticipated joy for going to the Promised Land. I am sad about, and stumbling over, the departure.

There is nothing but upside for my destination. No reason to not have a preference to be there. Yet, saying goodbye knowing you aren't coming back is emotionally racking.

There in is the challenge. That's why it's important to make lemonade today, and everyday going forward. I won't be back after I leave. I must find and express all the love I can before then, because that is what matters, and there are no second chances. There is no time to waste on all of the distractions of everything that can pull me off purpose.

There is living to do, God's beautiful bounty to appreciate, and people that must know how much I care, and how much difference they have made in my life. I must also try to make a difference to all that I can.

I doubt there is an easy way to say goodbye, for anyone that care and loves the amount that God has asked us to. There is no easy final departure, but accomplishing the right goals before you leave is a good departure and a right departure.

May God give us all the wisdom to appreciate his good works, share our love and be loved in the time we have.

Monday, December 16, 2013 – More Blessings Abound

"Reflect upon your present blessings, of which every man has many – not on your past misfortunes, of which all men have some." - Charles Dickens

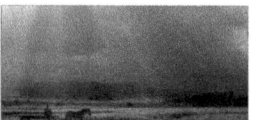

Thanksgiving is over, and Christmas is near. They of course are both rooted in separate central celebration goals, but to me they have one major feature shared, they celebrate family and friends too. Less so for Thanksgiving, but certainly with Christmas - the focus from the central idea is often lost.

Christmas is not a celebration of gift giving. While the main reasons we have the custom of giving and receiving presents at Christmas is to remind us of the presents given to Jesus by the Wise Men: Frankincense, Gold and Myrrh, it is not the point. Christmas is the celebration of the birth of Jesus. The reason the Christian world celebrates it, is that it He represents your salvation to the kingdom of God. Which makes him more important than any human that ever lived.

Even before Christmas we now see black Friday, and cyber Monday, and forever on with commercialized hysteria to lure you into gift giving. People measure the love for another by the value they pay for gifts. Others measure the status by what they receive. Its all fun to do, its great to please others, especially the kids, but the true meaning of Christmas has taken a distant row of seating to what is frequently an ostentatious display of opulence.

My Christmas wish is for everyone to think about the gift from God that comes in the form of forgiveness through the sacrifice of his only son who only asks for you to believe. In exchange for that, God offers an eternity of living in a perfect environment. How simple. How beautiful.

If you took away dollars from this year's Christmas, would you find more joy? Would there be more focus on the ones you love? Would you find any more gratitude for the sacrifice that Jesus made for everyone that believes?

In the end, the spirit of Christmas is about the love we share for each other, which includes family friends, neighbors and God. It's a time to humbly appreciate the amazing gift that God offers to all who believe. It's a time to show respect for the value of that act of love by graciously showing our love to others. It's a time to bow our heads and give thanks for the abundance of care and comfort that comes from God. It is also a time to give thanks to all of the blessing that we all so richly enjoy.

We know the world is not a perfect place, we also know that God has that planned for later. But as imperfect as this world is, I have found the blessings I receive to be amazingly abundant and richly rewarding.

I don't know what is down the road for me. This may be my last Christmas. It inspires me to want everyone to think about what is really important and hope they find the love and spirit of Christmas driving them to the true meaning and the most rewarding outcome.

God's Blessings, and Merry Christmas to all.

Monday, January 6, 2014 - Cancer - you do your Worst, I'll do my Best

"We will have no truce or parley with you, or the grisly gang who work your wicked will. You do your worst - and we will do our best. Perhaps it may be our turn soon; perhaps it may be our turn now." - Winston S. Churchill

The greatest moments of consternation in my life have been provided by cancer. Deep gut straining anxiety over what will happen, what to do, and what the impact will be to myself and to those around me. Moments just before sleep when you reach for answers, 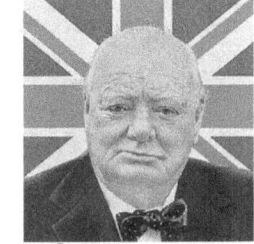 *that aren't there. For over three years and now entering the sixth round of the battle for my life, there have been plenty of those nights.*

Among many other factors, the anxiety of cancer is fueled by uncertainty, creating what seems to be mental cruelty, over having to wait and wonder what the outcome of a test or procedure will be. If that isn't enough, after a procedure, there is worry for how or if you are healing. Everything you don't understand can be scary. The quality of life and even the continuation of your life are at risk as you wait. Survival is our strongest instinct, so the tension created is strong. Experience and empathy internally aggravate those feelings, nearly to the same extent as your own, by reading the blogs of others that are going through the same things. Not because it impacts us directly, instead because all of us in the cancer ranks vividly relive what they feel, and are as frustrated and helpless to help them, as others are to help us. Nevertheless, we all continue to be engaged with each other, so that we may be supportive. We all understand the value of support; we have all received miraculous uplift from others that care.

Part of the angst we suffer is centered on the lack of control. We have no way to influence a positive result. In all my previous life outside of cancer, when the outcome of anything was important to me, there was always something I could do to improve the odds toward a favorable outcome. But it is not so with cancer. Cancer has dominant control, and there is very little we can do besides following the orders of the medical team in hopes of improving the situation or risk, and staying positive of course.

There are many treatments for cancer but precious few cures. Yet, I have one powerful armament, which can be found in my mind. In a word, it is faith. For clarity, in the end, unless a miracle cure emerges, cancer will kill me. But I don't worry about it or feel anxious very much anymore. Although, I think it would be inhuman to not worry some. At times I have caught myself during my darkest moments, when my guts literarily hurt from tension anxiety, and I will remind myself of the faith I have in God. The day I discovered I have cancer, over three years ago, I prayed to let God know cancer was too much for me to handle, and that he has the lead, I will follow. From time to time I forget and worry. Each time I then remember, and I am blessed with relief. A solution always emerges. Even though I have written about this more than once, it's always amazing.

However, there are a couple of new points I want to make. I am reminded of what an important decision having faith in God has been for me, especially as I watch others struggling with the same cancer fears. The one thing I wish I could broadly give away is faith in God. I am lucky enough to know it, I feel it, and am greatly comforted by it. It is free to everyone; yet it is impossible to give to anyone. You have to ask for it, you have to believe it. It is an individual choice, just as God meant for it to be. For people without faith, I find great discomfort in watching them struggle senselessly when the solution waits. Ultimately knowing how others suffer, and how good the solution God offers is, just brings a different kind of misery to me.

When you have faith, cancer cannot conquer. I believe that the greatest opportunity for soul enriching growth comes from adversity, and not so much from pleasure. Adversity challenges the soul to seek balance, harmony and peace. Adversity in the context of God's wisdom, brings focus to what really matters in life. It exposes worldly pleasures as mostly vapor. I think the exception is love.

Churchill's observation is so correct for cancer. While cancer seeks to do its worst and destroy us, it also provokes the finest attributes to emerge from humanity. Patients gain and behave with wisdom. Caregivers and medical teams treat from their hearts first, but also draw upon skill, experience and knowledge. Communities such as SU2C rally to raise support for comfort, care, and fundamental research to end human suffering.

Cancer will do it's worst; for it is the nature of the beast. Yet, individuals and humanity will do their best to seek ways to cope with, and hopefully soon, find a way to end this malady of human suffering forever.

Cancer has made me physically quite ill, but if the evil intent is to destroy me, then it has failed by every measure. It has been a pathway to experience important lessons that God teaches. My soul has richly profited from cancer. In measures that cannot be counted and with benefits that stretch to eternity. None of which would have happened without faith.

Round six begins on Wednesday January 8, 2014.

Cancer, you do your worst, and I will do my best.

I vigorously pray that everyone touched by cancer, also finds the love and wisdom of God, to hold in their hearts, so they may be comforted from their faith and know that all is well forever.

Tuesday, January 14, 2014 - The Bottom of the Pit is Where Real Character is Found

"The real character of a man is discovered not by what comes easy, but from what is most difficult."
– Randy Chalfant

The greatest virtues appreciated in human character don't come from the amusements in life. They teach very little. However, amusements and various other pleasures are good to be sure. I am thankful for all of the fun and joyful moments that I have been so richly blessed with throughout my life. I am thankful for the many moments that seemed difficult for some, from which I was also able to find joy anyway.

But I am not sure when we remember a person from the past, that we place high among the accolades and the score of character, an individual's joyful demeanor. The laughter they shared or created (unless they were a comedian) or the pleasures they pursued (unless they were corrupt) aren't counted much.

In the pursuit of human accomplishments society appreciates the fortitude of a person's ability to overcome great obstacles and show gritty determination to never give up. Winston Churchill, whom I greatly admire and have quoted frequently, led a nation to victory under seemingly impossible circumstances. Churchill spoke to the House of Commons as Prime Minister for the first time on 13

May, to announce the formation of the new administration:

"I would say to the House, as I said to those who have joined this Government: I have nothing to offer but blood, toil, tears and sweat." The peroration is perhaps the best-known part of that speech, and is widely held to be one of Churchill's finest oratorical moments. "Even though large tracts of Europe and many old and famous States have fallen or may fall into the grip of the Gestapo and all the odious apparatus of Nazi rule, we shall not flag or fail. We shall go on to the end. We shall fight in France, we shall fight on the seas and oceans, we shall fight with growing confidence and growing strength in the air, we shall defend our island, whatever the cost may be. We shall fight on the beaches, we shall fight on the landing grounds, we shall fight in the fields and in the streets, we shall fight in the hills; we shall never surrender, and if, which I do not for a moment believe, this island or a large part of it were subjugated and starving, then our Empire beyond the seas, armed and guarded by the British Fleet, would carry on the struggle, until, in God's good time, the New World, with all its power and might, steps forth to the rescue and the liberation of the old." Later he also said, "Never, never, never give up."

Society loves this resolve and gutsy determination. Big victories are bourn from exactly this type of thinking. Battling without this type of focus dramatically reduces the odds of obtaining a victory.

It doesn't matter what the unknowns are; we must fight. In fact, it is perhaps because of the unknowns that we must fight. That is what the brave do.

Yet, I doubt there is a single sane leader or individual that doesn't consider the realities of circumstances when their quite moments allow. It is hard to imagine that good reasoning can exclude rational consideration for all influencing circumstances.

A warrior is not recognized for the times they are gripped by fear, they all are. They are not recognized when they have had their fill and don't want anymore of it, they all do. Strangely, a warrior is honored because of the gripping fear, and because they find what it takes to go fight another day, and because they suffer, but do not complain. They don't complain because their dedication to a cause is greater than their personal discomforts or suffering.

John F. Kennedy summarized this when he said; "When the going gets tough, the tough get going."

After three years of fighting cancer, and now sure that I am no farther ahead than I was at the beginning, I am finding myself at the bottom of a pit looking up. I know there is light at the top. I know I cannot survive by simply starring up. I can only survive by continuing the struggle to climb. God has given me the opportunity to experience the type of circumstance that can only be sustained by the greatest resolve and determination. In the end, nobody will count the anguish, as the accomplishment if that is all that is experienced or expressed. Yet it is because of anguish, that perseverance and commitment to fight brings admiration. Not just for me, but for all that have ever been in this situation.

I feel stuck, I don't like it, I don't want it, I would like for it to stop, and so did every other soul in similar circumstances. Which makes me nobody special.

I'm not exaggerating when I say this is tough. But then so am I. This pit is deep and the climb is difficult, but it is for that very reason, that I have gained insights and character.

God never makes the challenge larger than the strength you have to persevere.

Gifts don't always come with ribbons, and the tough never quit.

Wednesday, January 15, 2014 - The Sunset Doesn't Last Forever

"The secret to a rich life has more beginnings than endings." - Reader's Digest

My battle with cancer is now three and a half years long. It has been a constant engagement, and I think it is fair to say that I have measurable battle fatigue and damage.

Monday I had a PET scan, today is Wednesday and Bonnie and I just left Sam's office. The PET really isn't remarkably different than what we saw three and a half years ago. But there in is the problem. Three and a half years of chemo and radiation have yielded no progress. Disappointingly, the cancer in my rectum is back, which means the radiation treatment wasn't effective and all of the pain was for not. Cancer in my lungs is making progress. Time to start chemo again in an effort to check the onslaught of the progression of this disease.

The challenging part is that when you start the cancer journey, you are more or less at the top of your physical ability. Once cancer starts, along with treatment, it is much like a ski slope that goes down a mountain. Except in this case the slope is related to physical abilities. It just keeps going down. When I first started this, I was at the top of the slope. When I start Chemo again next week, I will be starting from near the bottom, which means I will just continue to feel much worse.

Today was the first time that Sam brought up the end of life conversation. I'm not eminently dying here folks. But the distance to that horizon is considerably shorter from where it was when I started on this journey. There will come a time when the disease will simply kill me, or I will have to decide that the quality of life is just gone, and stop taking treatments.

Thus the realities of cancer are sneaking up on me.

As so many have dispassionately pointed out, we all have to go sometime. Watching the beautiful sunset doesn't last forever. However, to me it's personal. I haven't spent the last three and a half years with indifferent observation. My time has been spent gleaning out the values which have provided the space for me to experience so much that is good from so many of you. Spiritual awakening is priceless. I would never want to trade or take back any of that.

I have given a lot of thought to an end game since the beginning of this journey; today it feels like I am one step closer. I am feeling sadness in knowing there will be a goodbye in the future, I am also feeling excited for what awaits. I am certainly not looking forward to the illness of chemo!

The circle of life is an endless loop. My time is not over, just more valuable.

Round 6

The battle continues as I begin chemo again soon for round 6. The big difference now is that I don't see an end to treatment, unless the miracle drug is found.

Chapter 7 - God, Family and Friends

"Eternity is forever, you can only take the love given and taken from here." - *Randy Chalfant*

By now you realize that my journey was not made alone. In fact I believe the most important part of the experience is that it was about lots of people.

It would have been very easy to believe it was all about me. After all there is a great and demanding focus on the things that are going on with my body. But it doesn't take long to see that the circle of people that care for you is much larger and more important than that. You may be the catalyst to the activity, but the circle is larger and more important than you alone. Your leadership will set the tone for how you and the circle of relationships will feel about you and the disease. You can and should be honest with everyone - you don't have to gloss it, but the disease doesn't have to define you or your life either.

Remember also, there is far more respect from your circle for living through the disease, than from suffering from it.

It may be hard to face the music yourself, and even more difficult to tell others. But hiding it doesn't really make you stronger, or even appear to be strong. Hiding it from the people that care from you can present an image of fear and denial. It also denies others the ability to offer their care, which they will naturally want and in many cases need to do.

Faith in God

Bluntly, my well-being boils down to faith in a number of areas. First in God – it is critical to believe that you are in good hands and that the plan makes sense. Not that I think the plan may be reveled. Because that is not God's way most of the time, God is subtle. In Isaiah 7:9 God says "if you do not stand firm in your faith, you will not stand at all".

So, have faith. "For we live by faith, not by sight." 2Co5:7

You can't see it or touch it; you just have to believe it.

In your heart believe all will be well. I turned the outcome of this over to God, by Faith - from the very beginning. That has had a huge value in stress reduction to me. As I am relaxed, so are people around me.

God loves you more than you can measure. So, have faith that the right things are happening for the right reasons. I will say again, in the backdrop of eternity, the period of time you are battling cancer is nothing. It has been truly amazing to watch all of the challenges that have come up - the fear and consternation they have caused - and how each have been resolved through prayer. So many things have been solved in such handsome fashion, that we feel God has gone above and beyond the call.

With cancer, the opportunity is to experience all the love and care that surrounds you from the circle of people that are close to you.

That loving energy is enough to sustain you in your spirit and allows you to find the joy and happiness offered in life. Cancer and treatment is not the joy; it is what is enabled because of cancer that is joyful. Find it, and savor it, because it comes from the spirit of God, the love and generosity of humanity - and that is the only lasting and meaningful joy there is.

The Medical Team

From a medical point of view, I have had a terrific team. That is a critically important aspect of this. Just like God, you have to believe and have faith in the medical team.

Because of the care and concern of so many friends, especially early on, I received numerous recommendations to seek out various well-known cancer care centers. All of the recommendations were good, and all of the care centers were excellent.

But at the end of the day, I believe in Dr. Sam Shelanski. I have faith in him. I believe he is up on all of the latest and greatest cancer treatments, I believe he is current on statistical probabilities for outcomes based on cancer types and treatment regimen scenarios. I believe I am getting what has statically been proven to be the best approach. And I believe Sam cares for me and is committed to do what is right to keep me alive and as well as possible.

If I didn't believe that, I would search until I found someone I did have faith in.

Since I have found Sam, I am not on the Internet constantly, searching and researching my problems. I don't have enough time or energy to be Sam. He has lots of years of training and experience invested, there is no way I can catch up with that now to credibly take charge, and since I have faith in Sam, I trust him to be doing the very best for me that can be done. That relaxes me greatly and removes the burden of worry.

In addition, in the infusion center, nurses Alice, Brenda, Kim, Kathy, Julie, and Kait genuinely care.

In some ways I feel sorry for them. They are in the infusion center to provide patient care, but unfortunately the methodology for doing that is to administer copious amounts of what feels like poison. Seems like a conundrum that has to be tough on them. Yet, I love them too. They are kind, compassionate, and caring.

They see the administration of chemo as a path to helping to improve the probabilities of survival for the patient, and hopefully improve what life can bring to them.

Things can go wrong when you are taking chemo, and they watch it like a hawk. I can't overstate that. They are just fully engaged. As a matter of practice, they check, and cross check EVERYTHING. I know they are doing it right, I have faith in them too, and I can relax while I'm there, and take the chemo punishment without fear.

I just want to share a funny experience. Near the end of the first round of cancer, when things were in retreat, Sam decided to double-down on the treatment regime to make sure we were really kicking cancer hard.

Sam changed the chemo cocktail from "Full Fury" to "Full Fox Fury." That translates to dropping Camptosar and adding "Oxaliplatin" which is a really difficult chemo drug to endure, with lots of lousy side effects. As a result, they were carefully watching me to see how I would tolerate the initial infusion.

Within about 15 minutes of the start of the infusion, I began to have chest pains, where my heart is located. They told me if I felt anything unusual to let them know. So, I told Alice I was having chest pains. After about 5 minutes, she said she thought Sam should know, and went to tell him. Within about 90 seconds, Sam shows up – standing right in front of me, hands on his hips, he looks down at me and says, "Are you whining again"? Even though I was really ill, it was hysterical. It's great to be able to find humor in the middle of tough times - it just elevates my spirit.

Thanks Sam, Alice, Brenda, Kim, Kathy, Julie and Kait – I love you too!

> I followed Sam to a new health provider, so now I must include thanks to: Sam, Julie, Kate, Alan, Cathy, Jennifer, Shawna, Monica, Terry, Jennifer, Vanessa, Dr. Ceilley, Brad, Cindy, Deb, Brigid, and Both doctor Frank's.

Family

What relationship is closer than family? What humans can possibly care more?

To the patient, the onset of cancer is of course a really scary proposition. The possibility of a nasty disease, the horrifying stories of cancer treatment, and then you die; mentality is frightening to your very core as an initial reaction.

But, getting self-absorbed with all of that is unfair to the family that loves and cares about you. Don't think they don't know the same things you do, or aren't feeling the same degree of fear because they most certainly are. In some ways it may be worse. After all, if you die, you can look forward to heaven if you are a believer. On the other hand, your family just sees you as permanently gone.

In my case, I am the breadwinner, which can bring additional fear for the family if you are gone. But regardless of who you are in the family structure, it is lousy to think of anyone in the family going through cancer.

However, time and faith have a way of settling things. Bonnie and I have prayed and thought this through carefully. Everything that can be done to prepare from a support infrastructure point of view, has been done. So, from a business point of view, we worked though all of that, and just took care of it.

What is left is the emotional side of this. The only thing left after thinking through the impact of cancer that is important, is faith in God and the love we have for each other.

If God's plan is for you to die, then you are going to die. That definitely means permanent separation here on Earth. That is nothing new. The process has gone on since the beginning of time. It will not change. The only thing left to do here, is to savor the joy of each day, and to be sure God and your family know how much you love them.

I don't focus on the sorrow of death. I focus on the joy that life brings each day, and it is easy to find if you are true in your heart and are looking for it.

I feel my wife Bonnie, my son David, and my daughter Marci; look at it the same way. We have not had long teary sessions of regret. We have had lots of holidays, and other time together where things are family business as usual, with maybe a bit more effort in enjoying the time we do have. Perfect.

Of course there are sisters and brothers, in-laws, cousins, and so on. All of them care as well, and check-in, vying for quality time. Perfect.

Cancer has accelerated the desire to connect and enjoy time together.

Friends

Prior to cancer, I was just too full of myself to understand the depth of human compassion that comes from friends. I never could have predicted how many people would rise to express their concern and care for me.

Unless you are really tuned in, a living person may never see that. It seems we most often hear about the impact we have had on others as a eulogy while attending a funeral. How blessed and fortunate I am to have experienced it while still alive. If you have cancer you have the opportunity to experience it as well.

So many people have expressed how something I did for them had major value. Quite honestly, in many of their expressions of thanks, I couldn't remember that I had done anything.

That underscores one thing for me, as a normal part of being a fellow human; you have probably made contributions that have had significant impact on others. I can tell you it is a humbling experience to have friends come forward with expressions and sometime deep expressions of gratitude for your contribution. How would you know that stuff otherwise? I didn't!

But a brush with mortality will motivate people to let you know while they still can. It is an unbelievable and unexpected joy when it arrives.

Because of my global career, I have made friends all over the world. People that I feel connected to like I do family. People that care are concerned and want to express their care and their love.

Never underestimate the power and awe that friendships delivers. Nor the impact of sustaining you that friendships brings.

In my experience with cancer, that description fits most people. On the other extreme are people that just have too much personal difficulty dealing with your suffering. One dear friend I have, just won't communicate with me - period. He told me it is too much for him because of watching his sister die of cancer. That's OK. I get that.

Some people just don't know what to say. In the end, I find that it is not so important what you say as much as just letting someone know you care. Really, gifts and deep expressions of love are not necessary. Knowing someone cares is enough. It makes a difference.

For me, the expansive amount of love and support that came from so many people has been very uplifting. It just provided me with strength and the will to survive. In some ways I have felt a sense of responsibility to everyone to not let them down, I have wanted to not even expose them to any kind of grief. It made me feel I HAD to get better.

Friends have provided constant encouragement. It is hard to express how humbling that has been. It fills me with joy, energy, and the desire to live.

Truly, when your time comes, the only things that matter are the love you bring and have shared. The Lord Jesus commanded us to love our neighbors. Your friends do love you and from my experience – immensely!

There is no form of thank you that is large enough to adequately repay that.

Chapter 8 - Abundant Human Generosity

" Friendship improves happiness, and abates misery, by doubling our joys, and dividing our grief."

- Joseph Addison

Abundant human generosity, what an amazement it has been to me. What made so many people so good, and why was I blind to the largeness of it until recently? Maybe it is because I never really needed anything before now. I was always big and strong and able to attack anything I wanted.

Cancer changed that. I have become weak and fragile on the outside, yet stronger and better on the inside. An unpredictable yet welcome transformation. I would rationalize that becoming weaker physically would mean weaker mentally, but for me – that has not been the case. I have had major spiritual growth and am doing fine mentally.

Evidently the good nature of other people allowed them to know this long before I did. People, and I mean lots of them, arose to find ways to let me know they cared and that I mattered to them. Perhaps the nature of cancer in the past has most commonly denoted a death sentence in very unpleasant terms. Which is just not the case today based on technology improvements in fighting and winning cancer battles.

No matter – people care, and they want you to know they care. It is shared in so many ways. For some it is a call or an email. Others wanted to see me. Sometimes I have the strength to go have lunch or breakfast. Other times I don't have the health to go and sit in a restaurant. People knew how to solve that; they kindly called and asked permission to come to my house.

Some people were too far away to come over. They sent gifts. All sorts of things. Denny Yost sent very expensive steaks; Jamie Hurt once sent a bamboo plant, then a keyboard colon in a glass jar as a "backup colon" for me. Later, he then sent a model helicopter that I can fly around the house. My neighbor Pat Burnett sent outstanding chicken noodle soup. She then knitted a comforter for me. Wendy, her daughter, knitted a skullcap to keep my bald little head warm. My team at work sent a Sony PlayStation to keep me entertained.

Brian Bate offered to mow my yard.

I don't mean to slight anyone, but it is just a ridiculously long list of things people have sent to express their love and concern.

Beyond all of the gifts, the revelation to me was how many people could care so much and are so willing to take such extraordinary steps to insure I knew.

The hearts of these people are so large and so gracious that I am totally blown away. I have just never been the focus of such generosity. I have never seen it before in the ways that I see it now.

All of that spirit of generosity did not happen just because I happened to get cancer. I'm sure it was always there. I am just not sure why I was never aware that it was there or understood the breadth and nature of abundance it has. Who knew! I didn't!

Because of how good this spirit in people is, it has made my stodgy old value system collapse under its enormity. It has made me realize that my old thoughts of what was important were shallow as compared to the indescribable value and great good the generosity of others holds. Truly, it is in some ways embarrassing. On the other hand, I am grateful for the trumpeting wake up call.

I have found the loving kindness of friends to have a huge and unexpected impact on my psyche. I suspect that cancer patients in general experience this rallying call from many in their own relationship circles. It definitely had a profound impact on me.

I somehow felt the energy and it was healing and inspired renewed energy in me. I know that may sound a little hocus-pocus - nevertheless it is true. Maybe that is another example of the power of love. What a generous gift it turns out to be, and interestingly enough it was free. I doubt there is anything on the planet you can pay for that would provide the same value or health benefit.

Somehow people seem to know this and rise to the occasion. I am three and a half years into this battle now, and the human generosity is still going on.

Yesterday Kris Phillips called to set up a lunch for Bonnie and I, to meet with Dave and her. A dear friend from the Netherlands, Andreas Drenthen called yesterday because he saw in my blog that I am in remission again.

God please bless all of the kind people that have lifted me so far and for so long!

I know from my experience with cancer, that the majority of cancer patients I have been exposed to are upbeat, positive, and philosophically sound people. I found that to be a bit of a surprise. I expected people to be much further down in the dumps than they seem to actually be.

It seems that once you have gone through all of the initial shock, and have made it into a treatment regimen, that most people seem to adjust and somehow come to grips with the situation. They resolve the internal conflicts and reach something like a settled peace. That is an awe-inspiring testament to the good nature of people.

Yet, if you are reading this maybe you are still searching for resolution and peace or even just a commonality of experience. Perhaps you want to understand what you can do for someone that has cancer, or are having some other difficult health issue

First and foremost as a supporter, just be there. As minor as that may seem, it is huge in value.

For the cancer survivor, my advice is to be patient and pay attention to all that is going on around you. There are lots of wonderful people that want to help you. Medical teams that want to care and cure you. Your family wants you to be well. There are friends that care beyond reasonable measure, and are generous without bounds. Collectively, they create a nurturing and health-inspiring environment. Whether you will fully recover or not, you are in the cradle of the most loving environment you probably have ever experienced. Soak it in, it's good for you, and is a gift that can't be replaced.

It may seem that these things are not the solution to cancer, but in fact they really are. Cancer is cancer. It will rob you of health and it will change your life, as you knew it. You may get health back, or you may die. If you get your health back, hooray you win. If you don't, hooray you get the opportunity to experience God's grace, and the love that family and friends share with you.

I believe the only measure God has in the accomplishments column is what love you gave, and what love you got. It seems that is the only points of value that comes from scripture. Love

God, love your family, love your friends, and love your neighbors.

Love; it's what makes the world go around and cancer is a major catalyst to experience the power of it.

Beyond that and from a personal point of view, I have not focused on the multitude of issues I experience daily. After all, I have cancer, which creates functional issues. I have taken a lot of chemo, which feels like nothing short of mega poisoning, in addition to radiation. Together, they have created a long list of issues I get to experience daily. There have been a lot of books written that detail all of that. My view is so what, what did you expect?

My preference is to focus on the prize and the gifts. The prize is hearing your doctor tell you are in remission or if you are lucky you are cancer free! The gifts are all of your fabulous supporters that will pour their hearts out to help you and energize you.

The greatest gift of all for me has been the spiritual awakening. Just like all the incredibly generous friends that were lying in wait to ambush me with huge amounts of loving support, which I was previously unaware of, God was waiting too for me to wake up to his loving presence. I have read his book and have a much better and clearer view of that too.

On a personal note however, I must say that after reading the entire Bible, I now feel biblically illiterate. I should have spent the last thirty years working on understanding the richness of God's word. So for now, I need to play catch up. It also brings great hope and comfort to me.

Chapter 9 - The Lord's Contribution

"One person gives freely, yet gains even more;
another withholds unduly, but comes to poverty.

A generous person will prosper; whoever refreshes
others will be refreshed."   *- Proverbs 11:24-25*

No matter what, your best days are ahead.
Although, I would never trade my past.
Experiences have taught me to be who I am.

Perhaps everyone has a unique relationship
with the All Mighty. It's hard for me to know.
Anyone that does have faith and is a believer
probably feels special in that regard. I definitely
feel blessed. It's a long and personal story, but I
feel like I was literally touched by God when I was
a teenager. It was a very profound experience for
me then and even now. But as ignorance would
have it, I did not use it as the inspiration to follow
a life of a Pastor or some other God serving
profession.

In fact, I couldn't seem to find a way to really
serve God at all. I did go though the study
necessary to become a Christian and a member of
the Lutheran Church. But after I did that I just
didn't follow a church and frankly didn't much
care.

While saying that, I can also say that I have
always maintained a strong belief in God and have
tried to lead a good life, which for the most part I

believe I have. Along the way I have experienced the voice of the Holy Spirit of God in various ways. Some have been somewhat prophetic, like predicting the birth of both my son and daughter ahead of any real evidence. I don't know why these things were shared with me, but it was cool to experience.

God must have had this plan from the beginning it seems. As an example, years ago I was living in Texas and was on a business trip in San Francisco bay area. I was heading back to the airport on 101. Back then it had three lanes in each direction, and had no center barrier. I was in the fast lane driving 65 MPH and was late to the airport. It was then I heard the voice say to me, "SLOW DOWN AND GET INTO THE CENTER LANE." In my arrogant way, I mentally replied, " I can't I'm late and have to catch a plane". To which the voice more emphatically responded, "SLOW DOWN AND GET INTO THE CENTER LANE." So, I mentally replied, "OK FINE," So I hit the blinker checked the lane, let off the accelerator, and moved into the center lane.

Just as I had finished the lane change, BOOM! The front left tire blew; chucks of tire actually hit the windshield. When the rim hit the pavement, the car swerved hard to the left and I entered the left lane uncontrollably. If I had been in the left lane when that tire blew, I would have gone into the center medium that separates on-coming traffic, which would have likely put me into a head-on crash. God saved my knucklehead that day. Why? Because he had plans for me later.

Perhaps God got tired of my lack of attention over the years. Now and especially after reading all the scriptures, I know that God rejoices in the return of any lamb that has wandered from the herd. Maybe that is how he saw me. I feel that God never ignored me, even though I was not giving my fair share back.

What better inspiration does one need to listen-up to the divine calling that leads you back to the flock than to get cancer?

I'm telling you, a brush with mortality got my attention. The initial onset of cancer shook me to my soul with trepidation and doubt. Who do you turn to? Of course Bonnie was there, but she could not answer some of the larger questions for what the future looked like for me or us.

God is the answer. Who knows, it may even be a bit humorous for God; "Gee, Randy seems to have wandered too far and for too long. Hmmm? Let's try cancer to see if that will bring him back." Ok, I have cancer. I came running back like a scalded dog. Great that worked! – chuckles.

On a more serious note, it is impossible from this position to know what the playbook looked like. At the end of the day, I have never really thought that God caused the cancer as much as it just happened. A concept along the lines of free will. Truly it doesn't matter to me whether it was intentional or like a river flowing willy-nilly. What is important is that I got the call and answered it.

There is no measure to the value this experience with cancer has provided. I had never really lost my faith or belief; it just hadn't been an active part of my daily thinking. Now, God and the love of the people around me are a primary focus in my life. I pray multiple times during the day and rarely for myself but much more for the good outcome of others. That is largely due to the lessons I've learned through the experiences I've shared about human generosity. I have received and am now in debt to all that have carried me.

But to understand how much I owed, I felt like I needed the wisdom that God has given us, which is abundantly rich and clear in the Word of God. I am certainly not an expert on the Bible. If anything I am a neophyte. Even so, through the experience of cancer, the words, ideas, and concepts I have read in my study Bibles have leapt off the pages and into my soul. It is a shame that I could not have understood the power of it before. It may also be that I could not have understood the way I do now without life's experiences to measure and understand the Word. I probably would have had little appreciation. Again, it's hard to know for certain.

Whatever the case may be, now, I am humbled and grateful to my very soul.

In understanding the essence of the Bible, we all know that God never has cared about all of the things of prestige that I built and worked after. None of the things I own and have collected ever did matter. In fact, Jesus view was that it would be harder for a rich man to get to heaven than it would be to thread a camel though the eye of a needle, which more or less sums it up.

The measure of success on the eternal scale is what love you have in your mind and in your heart; based on the life you have lead as evidenced by your works and deeds.

There is nothing that could be more valuable for me to know. Everything else is now immaterial. I may have never figured that out, without the help of cancer. Which is why I have said that it may very well be the best thing that has ever happened to me outside of finding Bonnie. It may be the difference between having an eternal life in the sight of God, versus a far less desirable outcome.

I am therefore so grateful that life has worked out the way it has. I have had the experience of God's loving wake up call, the understanding of why it is so rich, a family that is as good as can be found, and friends that have carried me though some very difficult times.

Is there anything you can name that is more valuable than that?

Chapter 10 - Final Thoughts

"It's not whether you get knocked down, it's whether you get up."   *- Vince Lombardi*

It is my hope that you find some meaning for yourself in this book.

My intention more than anything else was to pay a debt forward for the loving attention and care given by so many.

It would be impossible to measure the influence this experience has had on me. The interaction with family and friends has helped to heal... at least for now. It has given me strength, energy and joy. It has given me a sense of fulfillment. It has made me feel like I matter. And it has been humbling to be sure, as I had no clue how many would rise to the occasion for me.

All of this came from caring people and most of it costing them nothing to let me know they care and that my cancer mattered to them. Yet, what that has given me is priceless. And it is what God measures as most valuable – which because of this experience I now know.

It is impossible to pay back all that has been given to me so generously. It has left me with only one option - pay it forward.

It is my deepest hope and prayer, the abundant good and joyful things that have happened to me, can be part of what you find in your experience with or near cancer.

My advice is that if you are focused on what is being taken away from you, look for what is being given. The gift of what is being freely offered is far richer that what is being taken away.

Your time may be near. Seek redemption and understand God's will if you care about eternal life. If you don't, please consider that the only chance you have for seeing your family again after you have died, is by the grace of God and his promise of eternal life.

I also believe all of the good works that are going around you are guided and influenced by God's guiding hand. Personally, I had a sense of responsibility and obligation to understand and act responsibly. Too me that meant I needed to read the Bible, and not just have my eyes pass over every word, but to in fact attempt to understand it.

If you have never done that – I strongly recommend you do. It is a rich gift of understanding so many things. If you already have, then you know what I am talking about. To be sure, one read is not enough. There is far too much in it to comprehend in one pass. Personally I am now studying every day.

There are many Podcasts from a variety of people also available. If you are too weak to read, listening is great too.

My prayers and best wishes are with all of you impacted by cancer. I am thankful and humbled to all that have helped to carry me this far. I am most thankful to God and our Lord Jesus Christ for bringing me back to the flock, and guiding everyone that has offered their care to me. It is impossible to repay – but I am thankful.

Best wishes, God's Blessings, and love to all of you.

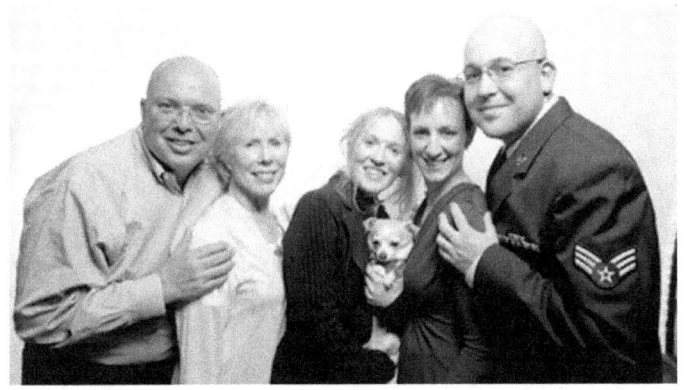

My Family - Randy, Bonnie, Marci, Kim, and David

The journey continues at:

www.randychalfant.com